Fitness Hacking

21 Power Tactics That Will Transform Your Workout Results

By Marc McLean

Author's Legal Disclaimer

This book is solely for informational and educational purposes and is not medical advice. Please consult a medical or health professional before you begin any new exercise, nutrition or supplementation programme, or if you have questions about your health.

Always put safety first when lifting weights in the gym. Any use of the information within this book is at the reader's discretion and risk. The author cannot be held responsible for any loss, claim or damage arising out of the use, or misuse, of the suggestions made, the failure to take medical advice, or for any related material from third party sources.

Photography by Victoria Murphy.

Table of Contents

RECOVERY AND HEALTH OPTIMISATION

MINDSET MASTERY

Introduction

Training hard in the gym, being consistent, eating like some sort of good food monk...but *still* getting nowhere?

Seeing small changes in your body, but not the lean muscle and fat loss the health magazines or the expensive PT promised you?

Been doing this whole gym thing for too long...everything you're supposed to be doing for way too long...yet feel like you're still a longgg way off reaching your fitness goals?

If you tick any of those boxes of frustration, you've picked up the right book. And you're about to get the right solution.

I'm already certain your problem is not laziness, a lack of trying, or an unwillingness to make serious changes in your lifestyle and diet. You've been doing the work to become a leaner, stronger, better version of yourself, and the fact you've bought this book proves it.

There's one core issue here.

One that few fitness nuts master.

And one that can be the difference between you absolutely smashing your fitness goals in less than three months...or crawling slowly for three years. (By which time you'll have cancelled your gym membership, eaten 3,247 takeaways, and punched yourself in the face a few too many times).

The key to you finally hitting your fitness goals is...<u>maximising your workouts through a series of highly effective FITNESS HACKS.</u>

Put plainly: most people only achieve a fraction of what's possible from their workouts because they've not optimised everything else.

Your one-hour gym session is only one part of the puzzle. There are lots of other fitness hacks I've discovered in more than 20 years of weight training - and being a health-obsessed nut – that can take your results to a whole new level.

They all add up to make a BIG difference over the course of any given week, and come under four key areas: fine tuning your workouts, a leftfield approach to nutrition for strength and performance, enhanced recovery, and mindset.

That's exactly why this book is split into four parts:

- Part One: Training Hacks
- Part Two: Nutrition Hacks
- Part Three: Optimising Your Recovery and Overall Health
- Part Four: Mindset Mastery

Each section is as important as the other, filled with individual lessons, top level tactics, and little-known adjustments you can start implementing immediately.

It's time to fast-track your fitness progress as I reveal the top hacks I've discovered in all these areas over the past two decades.

The book title, *Fitness Hacking*, might be interpreted that I'm giving you a shortcut to successfully achieving your fitness goals. This is partially true because it can potentially save you years of wasted effort on useless fad diets, or ineffective, complicated workout programmes.

But don't be mistaken in thinking what I teach is easy and less work. The fitness information in each chapter is easy to understand and straightforward enough to implement, but if you're looking for shortcuts, you're reading the wrong book.

As a fitness coach who specialises in weight training, this book is aimed at people who hit the gym. But there are a couple of chapters on training at home and outside without weights, while the sections on nutrition, recovery and mastering your mindset will arguably benefit anyone who works out.

Why should you listen to me? I've been involved in weight training for more than two decades, and have helped countless people achieve their fitness goals and become leaner, stronger, more confident versions of themselves.

My 'Strength Training 101' book series has reached more than 10,000 readers in under two years, and continues to reach new men and women every day, inspiring them to better themselves in and outside of the gym.

I'm also a fitness writer for leading websites such as Mind Body Green, and The Good Men Project, which have a combined 15 million+ visitors every month.

The book you're reading now is the sixth title in my Strength Training 101 series – and it's undoubtedly the best one yet.

While the other books lay out solid foundations for mastering weight training and have helped less experienced gym-goers build muscle, burn fat and become much more confident in the gym, Fitness Hacking takes things to the next level.

It comprises the best of the best knowledge I've learned for more lean muscle and less lard. It's packed with an unusual mixture of forward-thinking tactics that have been proven to help you become stronger physically, develop a rock-solid mindset, and improve your overall health and wellbeing.

Forget what you've read in 95% of the two-dimensional fitness books that are filled with the same boring bodybuilding advice, outdated nutritional plans, and complicated jargon that reads like a university textbook.

We're doing things differently around here. We always have. We're cutting out the crap - and we're going to have a laugh along the way.

The guidance and practices you'll find in this book are not simply what I've discovered through many years of research on weight training, sports nutrition, and the most effective routes to lean muscle, less fat and healthier lives.

No, everything I recommend is what I've implemented into my daily lifestyle, and what I've tried and tested when coaching men and women of all shapes, sizes, ages and abilities.

The hacks in Fitness Hacking work. And they can work big time for you. Even better, they are backed by science and I refer to various studies and sources throughout the book (and provide links at the end, because that's the kinda good dude I am).

They say that a picture says a thousand words. Well, a video must say closer to 10,000...and that's why I've also included bonus video demonstrations for free at the end of several chapters.

I want you and every single reader of Fitness Hacking to gain maximum benefit from this book, and I genuinely want to help you smash your fitness goals, no matter how many times you've failed before.

Want to know if what I teach works? Just check out the reviews of my other fitness books on Amazon, which have high average ratings, and have benefited people like you all over the world.

Now it's your turn.

This is the book that can finally end your fitness frustration. This is the very book that can help you develop muscle, strip away the unwanted fat, and become the strongest you've ever been physically – and mentally.

All you have to do is read – and then take action consistently.

Indecision, poor self-belief, and a lack of commitment hold too many people back from achieving their health and fitness goals. Don't be part of that flock.

Get up close and personal RIGHT NOW with the Fitness Hacks I'm about to reveal – so you can become the fittest, strongest, healthiest and best you that there's ever been.

TRAINING HACKS

CHAPTER ONE

Burn Fat On Autopilot By Manipulating Your Hormones

As I trudged down the hill panting, the sound of me gasping for breath was almost drowning out the Daft Punk tunes playing through my headphones.

It was 8am on an autumn morning and I'd returned to 'hospital hill' with my mates Paul and Nizzy. We all live near a hospital and next to it is a pretty steep hill where we'd meet up most Sunday mornings to do hill sprints.

If you know how punishing sprint training is, you'll realise it was a clever move choosing a hill so close to a hospital. #stretcheronstandby

On that particular day, things didn't exactly go to plan. As I got closer to the bottom of the hill after my second sprint, I heard a really loud sound roaring noise from behind me.

I turned around and my pal Nizzy was bent over with his hands on his knees spewing onto the tarmac.

He looked pale. He felt like crap. And he sounded like a cross between a broken hoover and a hyena.

I walked up the hill with the intention of asking if he was alright, or rubbing his back. Instead, I ended up staring directly into his puked-up breakfast lying in a hot, steaming mess on the road.

Moral of the story: don't be eating anything heavy before an intense workout, especially an early morning sprint training session.

But avoiding spewing is not the main purpose of this chapter, of course. It's all about the big benefits you can gain from exercising in the morning on an empty stomach.

I'm going to cover seven such benefits which should convince you that hitting the gym – or hill – without a belly full of breakfast is the way to go.

I'll also explain why training in a fasted state is a super hack for manipulating your hormones so that you can burn fat on autopilot, while developing muscle.

This is such an effective tactic that I completely switched to early morning workouts several years ago. Very rarely do I train in the evenings. This simple approach keeps me lean effortlessly, even when I'm enjoying takeaway meals at the weekend...occasionally followed by apple pie and custard.

I know morning gym sessions might not be possible for you due to work, kids, or the very close bond you have with your duvet. But it'll pay off if you can manage at least one morning workout on an empty stomach at weekends.

First, let's look at the importance of hormones in all of this.

Optimising Your Hormones For Efficient Fat Burning & Muscle Development

Too many people believe that burning fat and losing weight is all about calories in and calories out. There are many other factors, with one of the biggest being the functioning of our hormones.

Our standard Western diets filled with processed, junk food and typical eating patterns of breakfast, lunch, dinner - with snacks in between – has our hormones out of whack.

Two hormones that are key to the fat burning and muscle development process are: insulin and growth hormone.

I'll quickly go over each of them and demonstrate how training in a fasted state can manipulate these hormones in your favour. This will also make more sense as you go through the later chapters.

Insulin

This is a hormone that's released by the pancreas that allows your body to use glucose from carbohydrates in the food you eat for energy. Once there's glucose floating around in your bloodstream, insulin opens up the cells to allow glucose entry.

When there's excess glucose in the bloodstream, insulin encourages the storage of glycogen in the liver, muscle - and fat cells. It can also encourage the fat cells to store more free fatty acids and grow larger.

There are two ends of the spectrum when it comes to insulin: sensitivity and resistance.

Insulin resistance occurs when your body has been chronically overwhelmed with insulin repeatedly throughout the day that your cells stop responding properly to it. This is what happens with obesity and is linked directly to type 2 diabetes.

However, you can still have a level of insulin resistance without being obese or diabetic, and this will seriously hamper your efforts to lose bodyfat and get in great shape. Here's what happens in the body...

* Insulin resistance occurs due to overeating and poor dietary choices >> your cells malfunction and don't allow glucose entry >>

your pancreas overcompensates by producing even more insulin >> too much insulin turns off the fat burning switch in your body.

Now onto insulin sensitivity – the opposite end of spectrum. This is the realm of the athlete and where you can be through good nutrition and intermittent fasting.

When you're sensitive to insulin your body needs a smaller amount of the hormone to efficiently transport glucose into the cells. With less insulin secreted, you gain less weight – and your body's fat burning switch stays on.

Furthermore, when you do consume food it's going to be better absorbed into your muscle, fat and liver cells. This means your body will feel, look and function a whole lot better.

So you can see why it's important for your fitness goals – and your overall health – to improve your insulin sensitivity.

Growth hormone

This is another very important hormone because it is a key player in building muscle tissue and it also stimulates lipolysis (the breakdown of fats).

Another big benefit to growth hormone is that it's an antagonistic hormone to insulin. <u>When growth hormone levels are high, insulin is low</u>, and vice versa.

Levels of this anabolic hormone decrease naturally as we get older, but there are steps you can take to increase your body's production of growth hormone.

Lifting weights just happens to be one. Intermittent fasting is another, and I'll go into much more detail on a highly-effective method in a later chapter.

Bottom line: anything you can do to increase your growth hormone levels naturally through diet and exercise is a great move.

An extended break without food does it. A high-intensity workout does it.

An extended food break + high-intensity exercise = supercharged growth hormone levels.

Which takes me oh-so beautifully onto the...

Seven Superb Benefits Of Morning Workouts On An Empty Stomach

#1 You increase fat burning

When you bodyswerve breakfast and head straight to the gym you're already in a fasted state. You'll have been sleeping for around eight hours and, with another few hours at either side of eating dinner the previous evening and walking through the gym doors in the morning, you'll probably have been without food for between 10-14 hours.

Our bodies convert excess glucose from the food we eat to glycogen and this is stored as our main source of energy. However, when we go long periods without food our glycogen bank runs out.

What happens then? Your body turns to its fat stores to use this as fuel instead. Exactly what we want!

This ties in with my later chapter on intermittent fasting, where I go into more detail about the ideal fasting periods, and how you can stay lean without going on fad diets you'll end up hating.

My point right now is that combining fasting with exercise first thing in the morning can ramp up fat burning even more.

Lifting weights for 45 minutes, or completing a high-intensity circuit training session for example, requires a lot more coal in the fire. With glycogen levels low, that bodyfat at your belly, your ass, and wherever else you don't want it, becomes the coal supplier.

#2 Better performance because you don't feel bagged up/sluggish

Your body must divert some of its energy resources to the digestion process. That's why we always feel like taking a nap after a big Sunday roast, or feel zapped after our Christmas dinner.

Your body's main organs, including your liver, pancreas, and kidneys are all working overtime to help the food be broken down, processed and absorbed in your intestinal tract.

None of this comes into play when you exercise on an empty stomach. It means your body can focus its energy supply on the task at hand in the gym.

#3 You optimise the post-workout muscle development process

When you're working out hard with weights your body is temporarily in a catabolic (aka muscle breakdown) state. It's well known that when you have your post-workout meal or shake afterwards, the body switches from catabolic to anabolic (aka muscle building).

But what's barely known in the fitness world is that this post-workout anabolic phase is heightened after working out in a fasted state, such as in the morning.

A study, published in the European Journal of Applied Physiology, showed that muscle protein synthesis was improved.

Six young men took part in two experimental weight training sessions three weeks apart, which included exercises such as bench press, overhead press, leg press and bicep curls.

One workout involved eating a high carbohydrate breakfast 90 minutes beforehand, whereas in the other session they trained on an empty stomach after an overnight fast.

Blood tests and muscle biopsies were taken from each of the men one hour after training, and enzymes were analysed. It was shown that levels of 'p70s6k' were twice as high following the fasted gym session compared to training following breakfast.

This enzyme has a signalling role in the muscle building process and its elevation was interpreted as an indicator of muscle growth.

The research team also concluded that increased levels of p70s6k may lead to a quicker transportation of amino acids (the building blocks of protein) into muscle cells, which should result in a heightened anabolic response to your post-workout meal.

#4 You don't feel nauseous and have smoother workouts

If your body is struggling to break down a pre-workout meal, particularly if you have food sensitivities you may not be aware of, then sometimes it can leave you feeling nauseous.

And if your training partner or PT decides to put you through a monster session that day, you could find yourself looking for the nearest sick bucket.

I used to drink thick, sludgy protein shakes years ago before my gym workouts, and every time – without fail – I'd end up having a date with the toilet pan in the middle of my session.

I was drinking a brand that was laden with sweeteners and other ingredients my stomach clearly didn't agree with. It took me about six months before I figured out that the shakes were to blame for my stop-start interrupted workouts.

Of course, when you train on an empty stomach in the morning you don't have to deal with any of the above.

#5 It sets you up for an amazing day

Pushing yourself hard in the gym in the morning is the ultimate start to any day.

Some people find it a real struggle to exercise at any time of the day. Others find it a monumental task to even work out just once per week. So, to drag your ass out of bed and make it to the gym when most of the neighbours in your street are still sleeping will build your mental strength.

The rush of feel-good endorphins that exercise stimulates in the body is well-known, but I strongly believe that the mental benefits of training, particularly in the morning, are what really matters.

Not only are you testing yourself physically and developing strength, you're scoring a significant win at the beginning of your day. That winning theme, and feeling of accomplishment, will help put you in a positive mindset and vibration.

That early morning win will then have a knock-on effect on other areas of your life, such as your job, and in your interactions with people in your life.

#6 You're much more likely to maintain your workout programme

There are countless things that happen throughout your day that can distract you, or completely divert you away from your workout routine.

Having a stressful day at work, having to take your dog to the vet, the live football match on the TV at night.

When you make an excuse to skip the gym one day, it becomes easier to find another reason to miss the next session. A pattern slowly emerges...then suddenly you've only worked out twice in a fortnight.

The beauty of hitting the gym in the morning is that it's done and dusted - before anything else can get in your way. You're putting yourself first before anyone even has a chance to muck up your plans.

#7 It'll improve your sleep at night

I have some friends who like exercising after work because it helps them de-stress and sleep like a baby. At the same time, two or three past personal training clients have told me that they feel "wired" after exercising at night.

Their muscles may be tired, but their minds are buzzing with all the adrenaline after an intense workout. Sometimes that can make it difficult to nod off.

Shawn Stevenson, author of the book 'Sleep Smarter', recommends workouts in the morning to improve your sleep at night, and we'll be looking more closely at the morning workout/sleep relationship nearer the end of this book.

CHAPTER TWO

Quick, Efficient Gym Workouts For People Short Of Time

Want to be able to do a good weights workout, but just don't have the time?

Is 60 minutes, 50 minutes, or even 45 minutes in the gym too long for you most days?

I get it. When I worked as a reporter at my local newspaper around 15 years ago my boss fancied himself as more of a neurotic drill sergeant than an editor.

If we were 0.001 seconds over our 1-hour lunch break he'd know about it – and then he'd let you know all about it.

I used to enjoy going to the gym on my lunch break. It would help break up manic Mondays, or shitty Wednesdays, and I'd actually feel recharged in the afternoon after a good weights session.

Problem was, it would take me a minimum of 70 minutes each time (50 minutes workout + 20 mins round trip travelling to and from my local gym). Then I'd be sneakily trying to eat my lunch at my desk when I was supposed to be typing up a court report for the newspaper, or calling the police to get some pointless story about tools being stolen from someone's garden shed.

I needed to change things up to avoid groans from my boss or, even worse, the silent treatment and a terrible atmosphere in the office all afternoon.

I had two options: go to the gym after work or find a way to shorten my time in the gym.

I immediately felt resistance to the gym after work idea. My brain instantly said: "No chance!"

The gym was always sooo busy between 5pm and 7pm, and quite often the dumbbells I wanted were being used by somebody else, or some teenager would be hogging the cable machine for 20 mins.

Did I say 20 mins? I meant, he'd actually be on the cable machine for approximately two minutes - and just standing around in front of it looking at his mobile phone for 18 minutes.

I don't know about you, but after a long day at work the idea of sitting down on my sofa rather than a weights bench is a much more appealing option.

For some people it's the opposite. Especially if they want to delay seeing their wife or husband's face for another hour or two.

Okay, back to the choice I had to make: gym after work...or somehow shorten my workouts?

It was obviously the latter and, at the very moment I decided this, God struck my cranium with a lightning bolt of delightful wisdom.

Why? Because I instantly figured out how to shorten my workouts in five words: DROP SETS and SUPER SETS.

These are ultra-efficient training systems you can apply to any weight training session that can literally cut your workout time in half.

Goodbye 1-hour sweaty gym sessions. Hello 30-minute extra sweaty gym sessions.

Yes, while drop sets and super sets make for short, effective workouts. They also turn up the intensity a notch or three.

My friend Ross had introduced me to drop sets a couple of years earlier. We were training together for the first time and I was expecting we'd simply choose an exercise, he'd do one set, and then I'd do the next set while he had a rest, and so on.

It didn't quite work out like that. We started with bench press and after Ross did his first set, he looked up at me from the bench and said: "Can you take 20kg off mate?"

So I pulled a 10kg disc off each side of the barbell, slid the safety collars back on, and within seconds he was hard at it again; lowering the bar to his chest and pressing back up forcefully.

"Can you take off another 10kg," he said, looking up me after racking the bar again.

I took 5kg off each side, and Ross quickly smashed out a third set on the bench press.

This was all new to me because I was so used to always focusing on lifting heavy, and trying to increase the weight in subsequent sets where possible.

Decreasing the weight in sets two and three was never the done thing for me. It also goes against my "3,6,9 Training Principle" where I recommend gradually increasing the weight if you can comfortably manage 9 reps or more.

But I am a huge fan of drop sets and would argue that this system is equally effective as other weight training practices for muscle development and fat loss.

You might be thinking: "but if I'm decreasing the weight each time surely it's just going to be too easy?"

I wrongly thought that too.

Here's the big difference: *the lack of rest between each set works your cardiovascular system hard and fatigues the muscles effectively, despite the lighter amount of weight you're lifting.*

So while 'progressive overload' (aka gradually increasing the weight when your muscles get stronger) is the name of the game in the weight training world, drop sets is the exception.

You can still make great progress in muscle development and burning fat...and you can do it in less time. When training on your own, you can complete a solid weights workout in 30-40 minutes by following the drop sets system.

This means that lunchtime workouts are possible, if you have a gym nearby.

It means that you can blast out a great workout in the morning before work, and get fired up for the day ahead.

And it means that you can maintain your gym programme, whether you're a guy who works 167 hours per week, or you're a mum who thinks there's not enough hours in the day.

There is time. It's drop sets time. Now I'm going to quickly walk you through how I'd plan out a gym session using the drop sets system. Then I'll explain the similar super sets system.

This is just so you're clear on the ideal amount of exercises you should be doing, the optimal rest period between each set of exercises, and how much weight you should be lifting.

Drop Sets: The Basics

Exercises per workout: between 5 and 8. (If you do just 5 exercises you'll definitely be finished your gym session in under 30 mins).

Sets per exercise: 3.

Repetitions in each set: aim for between 6 and 9.

Rest period between each set: 20-30 secs (30 secs max).

Weight reduction after each set: around 25%.

Messing about between exercises, posting gym selfies on Instagram, wasting time watching Rita Ora music videos on the gym TV: 0.

Now let's put all of the above together into a typically-brilliant drop sets workout.

Quick note first: I strongly recommend using a gym training diary and planning out all your gym workouts in advance. Your results will improve dramatically with a gym training diary that'll keep you focused and on track.

Here's an example of a workout designed using a variety of highly-effective weight training exercises

Exercises: squats, deadlifts, bent over row, dumbbell press, upright row, barbell curls.

Remember, if you're unfamiliar with any of the exercises I talk about in this book, they're all covered in detail in my free Strength Training 101 exercises guide. (Download link included at the end of this chapter).

Workout example: squats 80kg/175lbs >> 20-30 secs rest/taking plates off the bar >> squats 60kg/130lbs >> 20-30 secs rest/taking plates off the bar >> squats 45kg/100lbs >> short rest and then set up the next exercise.

Deadlifts 90kg/200lbs >> 20-30 secs rest/taking plates off the bar >> deadlifts 65kg/145lbs 20-30 secs rest/taking plates off the bar >> deadlifts 50kg/110lbs >> short rest and then set up the next exercise.

Bent over row 40kg/90lbs >> 20-30 secs rest/taking plates off the bar >> bent over row 30kg/65lbs >> 20-30 secs rest/taking plates off the bar >> bent over row 22.5kg/50lbs >> short rest and then set up the next exercise.

No need for me to do the same for the rest of the exercises, I think you get the picture. The key here is starting with a fairly heavy weight: one where you can complete between 6 and 9 reps.

If you can comfortably complete more than 9 reps for that first set then the weight is too light. If you can barely manage six reps – with good technique of course – then the weight is too heavy.

If you're pretty new to weight training, then the first couple of drop sets workouts might be a bit experimental to see what weights level you're currently at. But you'll soon figure out your optimal weights level and you can adjust as you become stronger and more confident with the exercises.

Then you'll simply apply the drop sets fundamentals I've just covered:

- Begin set #1 of each exercise with an optimal weight where you can complete 6-9 reps.
- Drop the weight by 25% as soon as you've finished that initial set.
- Allow a maximum amount of 30 secs rest before starting set #2 with the reduced weight.
- Repeat the weight reduction and limited rest period before completing your third set.
- Move onto the next exercise in your programme (which you've listed in your gym training diary of course because you're a very organised individual and take heed of my fine advice).

Super Sets: Pairing Up Exercises

Exercises per workout: between 6 and 8.

Sets per exercise: 2-3.

Repetitions in each set: aim for between 6 and 9.

Rest period between each set: 20 secs (20 secs max).

Weight reduction: reduce usual weight by around 25% for each exercise due to intensity.

This is another quickfire style of training with little rest in between each set, but it involves pairing up different exercises. You would do exercise #1, take 20 secs rest, do exercise #2, take 20 secs rest, and then repeat.

For example, a planned super sets workout may look like this:

Pair 1: squats + bent over row (set 1 of squats >> 20 secs rest >> set 1 of bent over row >> 20 secs rest >> set 2 of squats >> 20 secs rest >> set 2 of bent over row).

Then take 1-2 mins rest to recover and set up the next pair of exercises.

Pair 2: military press + lat pulldown machine. (set 1 of military press >> 20 secs rest >> set 1 of lat pulldown machine >> 20 secs rest >> set 2 of military press >> 20 secs rest >> set 2 of lat pulldown machine).

Take 1-2 mins rest to recover and set up the third pair of exercises.

Pair 3: upright row + barbell curls. (set 1 of upright row >> 20 secs rest >> set 1 of barbell curls >> 20 secs rest >> set 2 of upright row >> 20 secs rest >> set 2 of barbell curls).

Take another 1-2 mins rest to recover and set up the final pair of exercises.

Pair 4: clean and press + cable row.

By doing these exercises in pairs, and with little rest in between, you can fly through a workout much quicker than you'd normally do.

The only downside is that this style of training is pretty intense and will really get the cardiovascular system going, therefore you'll have to drop your usual weight by around 25% in order to complete 6-9 reps of every exercise.

Some Final Pointers...

#1 Drops sets and super sets are awesome if you don't have a lot of time to spend in the gym, but always warm up for two or three minutes first before getting started.

Perhaps a bit longer if you're an older gym-goer, or haven't trained in a while. You don't want end up out of action for weeks or months with an injury just to save a few minutes on your overall gym time.

Do a light jog on the treadmill for 1-2 mins to get the blood flowing, and then do some basic stretches for your legs and upper body. It's a good idea to do some really light weight reps of exercises you plan on doing in that workout.

For example, if you're doing squats then do 5-6 reps with the bar only, or if you're doing dumbbell flyes then pick up weights that are 1/3 of what you'd usually lift and do 5-6 reps to help loosen up and prepare your muscles for what's to come.

#2 If you do have more time to spend in the gym than normal, then try something different to drop sets. Variety is good for shocking the muscles into growth and development.

#3 Good technique always comes first. Don't let your form slip on any of the exercises just to try and lift more weight. Doing exercises incorrectly is stupid – and can easily result in PAIN. (Said in Mr T's voice).

BONUS RESOURCES

- I've created a video on drop sets and super sets on my Weight Training Is The Way YouTube channel.

Quick Weight Training Workout …In Under 30 Mins:

https://www.youtube.com/watch?v=svsthHj9E5Q

- You can also download my Strength Training 101 Exercises Guide e-book for free at my website:

www.weighttrainingistheway.com/exercise-demos

CHAPTER 3

Quick Home Workouts For People Really Short On Time

One kettlebell, one rug, and my brand new Bose music speaker...

Those three items – and just four minutes - were all I needed for a great workout in my living room.

The new music speaker had just arrived in the post that morning and I couldn't wait to blast out tunes on it during my super-short, but super-intense, training session.

I connected my mobile phone to the speaker, flicked to my classic dance tracks playlist on Spotify, and then opened up the 'Tabata Timer' app on my mobile phone to set everything up.

"Prepare – 10 secs, Work – 20 secs, Rest – 10 secs, Cycles – 8."

Then it was time to get my Tabata workout started – and annoy the hell out of my neighbours with the music cranked right up.

Tabata training essentially involves 20 secs of exercise at maximum effort, followed by 10 secs rest, repeated for eight cycles/rounds. This short, sharp burst of training is over very quickly, but the high level of intensity elevates your metabolism, and maintains fat burning for up to 24 hours afterwards.

Tabata is a unique form of high-intensity interval training (HIIT) that was devised by Japanese scientist Dr Izumi Tabata. Back in 1996, he worked with the Japanese Olympic speed skating team and studied the effects of short bursts of extremely high exercise on the athletes.

A test was then carried out involving two groups of athletic men in their mid-20s on a stationary bike. The first group performed basic, steady exercise and pedaled on the bike at around 70% of their VO2 maximum; similar to a jog outside or on the treadmill.

The second group pedaled flat out at their maximum for 20 secs and then took 10 secs rest. This was repeated for eight rounds. Their effort equated to around 170% of their VO2 max in what was essentially 20 secs full-on sprints.

Both groups of men did their form of training five times per week, over a period of six weeks. The moderate-intensity group of men worked a total of five hours, while the high-intensity guys did just 20 mins overall.

The research found that the four-minute Tabata style of training had the same effects on aerobic performance improvement as 60 minutes of moderate-intensity exercise.

However, the Tabata group also saw a 28% improvement in their anaerobic capacity. (Anaerobic exercise is fueled by energy stores in your muscles, while aerobic exercise relies solely on oxygen).

So, not only is Tabata a much shorter workout, it's also more effective than longer, moderate exercise.

In this chapter we'll delve into why Tabata training can be beneficial for you, and how you can apply it at home if you don't want to go to the gym.

The biggest Tabata workout benefit is the most obvious one: it's over very quickly.

Five Fantastic Benefits Of Tabata Training

#1 It preserves muscle

One of the biggest drawbacks of longer, drawn-out cardio training is that it eats into hard-earned muscle tissue, aswell as burning fat.

Not so with the Tabata protocol, partly because of the short amount of time if takes to complete a Tabata session.

Also, the intense nature of working flat-out in a Tabata session places so much stress on the muscles that it signals your body to make more muscle tissue to compensate.

The result? Lower bodyfat levels, with lean muscle maintained.

#2 You keep burning fat long after you stop training

As mentioned earlier, this intense style of exercise is like a rocket to your metabolism – and that rocket can stay airborne for up to 24 hours, according to research.

Pushing yourself to your level 10 maximum capacity in Tabata training has "profound effects" on post-exercise metabolism, according to researchers at the Auburn University's Kinesiology Laboratory in Montgomery, Alabama.

They concluded that it would take FIVE times the amount of typical cardio exercise to shed the same amount of calories as you do in a four-minute Tabata.

How long does the post-workout burn last? Studies have shown anywhere from 4-24 hours. It all depends on the individual, level of effort, types of exercises involved etc.

One thing's for sure: four testing minutes of Tabata gives you plenty of bang for your buck!

#3 Anti-aging effects

Mitochondria are known as the powerhouses of cells, and they play a key role in metabolism and energy production. Mitochondrial dysfunction is an important part of various diseases associated with aging, which makes sense as your body's ability to produce mitochondria reduces with age.

However, research has shown that high-intensity interval training, such as the Tabata protocol, can trigger the creation of new mitochondria in your cells.

#4 It's straightforward (but not easy), cheap and efficient

There are no complications with Tabata training. It's simply a case of working out like crazy for 20 secs, followed by gasping for air for 10 secs, and then repeat.

It's also cheap because you don't need a gym membership or any fancy equipment to do a Tabata workout. There are a wide variety of bodyweight exercises you can do, as well as plenty others with basic pieces of equipment such as a kettlebell, dumbbells, skipping ropes etc.

It's efficient because you can roll out of bed in the morning, jump straight into it, and be done and dusted and in your shower within five minutes.

I've heard Tabata training being described as the "fastest way to get fit and lean". With a session done in as little as four minutes, there's no arguing with that.

But I don't think it should be your only way to get fit and lean, as a more substantial programme involving heavy weights will deliver best results.

Personally, I like to do a Tabata abs session at home on my rest days from the gym, or sometimes at the end of my weight training workouts to keep my stomach flat and in shape. This will involve four exercises completed twice in the usual '20 secs on, 10 secs off' Tabata style described earlier.

Tabata Abs Workout In Action

Put a mat on your living room floor, or use the rug, to make it more comfortable while doing the workout.

Choose four abs exercises that you can do one after the other, and you'll simply repeat them to complete your full 8 rounds.

Get the Tabata timer app set up on your mobile phone, punching in 'Prepare – 10 secs, Work – 20 secs, Rest – 10 secs, Cycles – 8'. There are plenty of free Tabata timer apps on the iTunes and Android stores that you can download to your phone.

Here's an example of a Tabata abs workout I like to do in the gym:

- 'Ankle slappers' – 20 secs work, followed by 10 secs rest.
- 'Spidermans' – 20 secs work, followed by 10 secs rest.
- 'Leg raises' – 20 secs work, followed by 10 secs rest.

- 'Russian twists' – 20 secs work, followed by 10 secs rest.
- Then repeat each of the exercises again in the same way.

A Tabata workout may sound and look easier than it really is. But we're not going for a stroll in the park...it's an all-out sprint during the exercise cycles. No messing around.

And once you become fitter and are breaking less sweat than usual, you can take it up a level by doing 12 cycles (4 exercises x 3 rounds).

Get to the stage where you can manage 12 comfortably? Feeling like a machine? Then why not step it up to 16 rounds? That means one full Tabata session with 8 cycles, have 1 minute rest in between, and then do another Tabata session afterwards – for a total of 16 rounds.

The fast-paced, highly-demanding nature of Tabata means that it'll take several weeks and months before people can think about doing more than one proper Tabata session.

I'd also recommend only doing it a couple of times per week, particularly if you're also doing other exercise during the week, to ensure your body recovers properly.

BONUS RESOURCES

- I've created a free Tabata training video demo for you on my Weight Training Is The Way YouTube channel.
- **Quick Home Workout...For People Really Short On Time:** https://www.youtube.com/watch?v=3FAs11raMZA&t

CHAPTER 4

How To Become A Chin-Up Champ

Anyone can pick up a couple of dumbbells and do some curls.

Anyone can lie on a bench and press some weight above their head.

And just about any human can jump on an exercise bike and get their sweat on.

But chin-ups? Proper chin-ups? That's a whole different ball game.

And pull-ups? Well, we're down to a select few people in most gyms who can rattle out a full set of this back-blasting exercise with excellent technique.

Chin-ups and pull-ups are arguably the best upper body exercises you can do. They blitz fat and develop solid muscle. They're a sign of true strength.

Yet so few people can do them.

In over 20 years of gym training, I've never witnessed any other effective exercise being completely body-swerved as much as I do with chin-ups.

I'll see guys wearing their gym gloves doing all sorts of fancy biceps exercises involving ropes, and dumbbells, and all sorts of contraptions.

I'll see others implementing the latest 'bulging biceps in 2 weeks' routine they've just read about in Men's Health magazine.

Meanwhile, a ball of tumbleweed is rolling past the tried and tested spot in the gym where the real results happen...the chin-up bar.

Chin-ups are hard as hell, I get it. And yes, pull-ups are even harder. But don't you want to be part of the elite crowd that dominates the toughest exercises that everyone else avoids?

Don't you want to feel ridiculously strong and in full charge of your body by conquering such a tough bodyweight exercise?

Don't you want to benefit from the full amazing effects one single movement can have on sculpting your torso, blitzing fat, and building your abs...all at the same time?

Yep, I thought so. The whole purpose of this chapter is to help you achieve exactly that.

The good news is that just about anyone can become a chin-up champ, or pull-up pro, even if doing one single rep seems impossible right now. I've helped many people through personal training become awesome at these awesome exercises, and achieve what they never thought was possible.

I'm talking about people of all shapes, ages and sizes. Yes, it may take longer if you're carrying a lot of excess weight but by gradually losing fat through weight training and developing your upper body strength simultaneously you can get there.

The bottom line: chin-ups and pull-ups are too damn effective to ignore. They're unquestionably among the best exercises for adding lean muscle, building strength, sculpting good muscle definition, and burning fat.

If you're serious about getting in great shape then it's time to start giving these exercises the attention they deserve.

The Difference Between Chin-Ups & Pull-Ups

Sometimes chin-ups are referred to as pull-ups, and vice versa. Don't know if it's an American thing...or if somebody was just mixing vodka instead of water with their protein powder when planning their workouts.

But there's two clear differences between these upper body exercises: how you grip the bar...and the muscles worked.

Chin-ups: underhand grip and hands at shoulder width. Muscles worked: biceps, latissimus dorsi, lower trapezius, forearms, and abs.

Pull-ups: overhand grip and hands at slightly wider than shoulder width. Muscles worked: shoulders, latissimus dorsi, trapezius, triceps, forearms, and abs.

The Right Way To Do Chin-Ups & Pull-Ups

If we're going to do this, we're going to do it right. No poor form, no half reps...and no injuries.

Chin-ups is definitely the easier of these two tough exercises so I'd always recommend focusing on mastering chin-ups first. Then you can build your upper body strength before moving onto pull-ups.

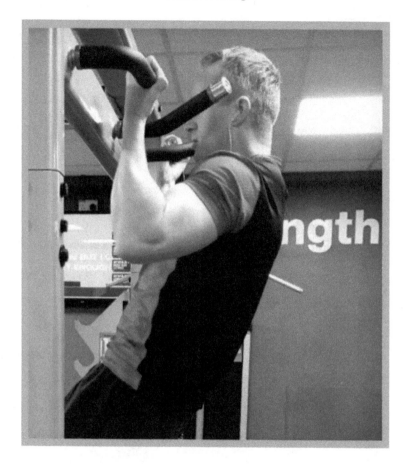

Chin-ups the RIGHT way...

Step 1: Grab the bar above your head at shoulder width with an underhand grip, which means your palms are facing towards you.

Step 2: Gripping the bar tightly, lift your feet off the group, cross your legs at the bottom, and begin in a dead-hang position.

Step 3: Pull your body upwards by squeezing the bar with your hands and engaging your upper body muscles and core. Continue to pull until your chin is over the bar.

Step 4: Slowly lower your body, maintaining a firm grip as you straighten your arms and return to the starting hanging position.

Chin-ups the WRONG way...

- Grabbing the bar with a wide grip: this will put strain on your shoulders and could lead to injury. Your hands should always grab the bar at shoulder width.
- Pulling yourself only halfway up: your chin should reach the bar and you should really feel the squeeze on your biceps.
- Not lowering your body enough as you come back down: this is only a half rep. Instead, you should lock your arms out at the elbow and drag yourself all the way back to the top.

Now onto pull-ups the RIGHT way...

Step 1: Grab a pull-up bar at slightly wider than shoulder width, with your palms facing away from you.

Step 2: Gripping the bar tightly, lift your feet off the ground and begin in a dead-hang position.

Step 3: Pull your body upwards by squeezing the bar with your hands and engaging your upper body muscles and core. Continue to pull until your chin is over the bar.

Step 4: Now slowly lower your body, maintaining a firm grip as you straighten your arms and return to the starting hanging position.

Pull-ups the WRONG way...

- Grabbing the bar at too narrow an angle. Remember to keep your hands at just slightly wider than shoulder width.
- Swinging/kicking your legs around as you pull upwards. Instead, focus on tightening your core/abs to help keep you steady.
- Jerking your upper body and head upwards to get your chin over the bar. Pull your arms fully until you reach the top for a proper repetition.
- Letting your body just drop to the bottom. This will likely cause an injury. Slowly lower yourself downwards.

How To Go From Rookie To Pro

It's one thing knowing the do's and don'ts of these awesome exercises, but it's another thing actually doing them.

My first attempt at doing pull-ups was an epic fail. I barely moved an inch, and so I just pretended I was hanging from the bar stretching. When I eventually let go 20 secs later I obviously had a quick look around to see if anyone had witnessed my glorious failure.

These days, I regularly do several sets of pull-ups and chin-ups with 25kg strapped to my waist. I'm not expecting you to put down this book on the spot and start clapping your hands (but do feel free). My point is that it doesn't matter if you can't complete a single rep, you absolutely can become a chin-up and pull-up pro.

I've seen plenty of clients master both proper chin-ups and pull-ups in as little as six weeks.

It just takes practice, perseverance, gradually building your upper body strength and becoming more comfortable with the technique.

I'll show you exactly how to do this step-by-step.

Stage 1: Assisted Repetitions

To progress towards achieving your first chin-up you must start by doing repetitions with assistance. There are two ways to do this: assisted machines or resistance bands.

Many gyms have machines that give you assistance when doing chin-ups, pull-ups and dips.

You rest your knees and shins on a cushion that compensates for some of your bodyweight. You can adjust how easy or difficult it is by altering the weight level on the machine.

- Step 1: Set the pin on the machine to a reasonable level, maybe around the halfway mark of the weights, and this will give you sufficient 'lift' when you do the exercise. Taller, heavier people may have to set the pin to a higher level for additional weight support.
- Step 2: Step up and rest your knees on the cushion, while grabbing the bar above your head.
- Step 3: Extend your arms until they're straight and then pull back upwards again. The cushion under your knees will give you a helping hand, pushing you as you rise.
- Step 4: Repeat this for as many reps as possible, always focusing on good technique as described earlier. Once you can comfortably manage 12 reps lower the weight setting on the machine, making it slightly more difficult, and again gradually work your way up to 12 reps.

If your gym doesn't have an assistance machine, resistance bands are a good alternative.

These provide support during the exercise, taking some of the bodyweight off you, making it easier to pull yourself up and lower yourself.

You can buy resistance bands fairly cheaply online from the Amazon website, and there are various thicknesses based on your strength and fitness. Beginners should at the very least go for the band with the medium thickness.

- Step 1: wrap the band around the bar/pull-up handles above your head.
- Step 2: Grab the band at the halfway point (not the bottom of the loop) and stretch it downwards.
- Step 3: Rest your knees inside the band for support, let it press against your shins, and then reach up to grab the bar.
- Step 4: Follow the directions given earlier for completing chin-ups and pull-ups with good technique.

Stage 2: Building Your Strength And Increasing Repetitions

The more you do these exercises the more your strength will grow. The aim should always be to progress in every workout, trying to do at least 1 more rep than the previous gym session.

I like to do 3 sets of chin-ups and pull-ups...and then count the total.So for example, if I complete 9 reps in my first set, then 7 in the next, and 6 in my last set, I'll mark the total 22 down in my gym training diary.

Next time I'm training I'm aiming to hit at least 23 reps over those 3 sets. This will keep your workouts exciting and challenging.

Finally, once you can do 12 good reps either at the lowest support setting on the machine, or with a thinner resistance band, you'll be much stronger.

Then it's time to move onto stage 3...doing proper unassisted reps.

Stage 3: Full Bodyweight Repetitions

You've been continually developing upper body strength. You've mastered the technique.

You're much more confident with chin-ups or pull-ups...

Now you're also ready to move onto working on doing unassisted reps and building upon these week after week.

Here's a three step process to do exactly that:

- Step 1: Start confidently and focus on that first single full rep.

When moving onto doing chin-ups or pull-ups without any assistance simply focus on perfecting the initial rep. You might manage just one, you might hit two or even three. But remember, most of the seven billion peeps on this planet cannot do these tough exercises at all so you're in a strong minority.

Let's just focus on getting that first single rep in the bag.

- Step 2: Forget everyone else in the gym.

Don't be self-conscious or worry about people watching you when working on your unassisted reps for the first time.

Firstly, a fair chunk of people in the gym won't be testing themselves as hard as you're about to. Let them trudge along on the treadmill getting nowhere.

Secondly, the other more experienced gym members will either be too busy concentrating on their own workout, or will genuinely be pleased to see you going for it.

I've always got massive respect for anyone really pushing their limits in the gym, no matter what stage they're at.

- Step 3: Compete with yourself.

Just like with the assistance machine, resistance bands, and your workouts in general, the aim should always be to keep making continual progress and trying to outdo your previous performance.

I always bang on about the importance of a gym training diary. A small notepad or digital notes app on your mobile phone will make a huge difference in keeping track of your gym workouts and push yourself harder.

If in your first week of doing unassisted chin-ups or pull-ups you managed two reps, mark that down in your training diary – and then try your hardest to go one better the following week. If you're working out three times per week then you've got three attempts at it.

The next week try to add another rep, and so on. Sometimes you might only equal the same number of reps as before. That's cool, but the key is to always keep challenging yourself to go one better.

Not only will this add an element of excitement to your workout and get your charged up for training, it'll make you stronger physically and mentally. Your confidence levels will also skyrocket when you start racking up gym performances you thought you never had in you!

This will obviously only spur you on more – and those reps numbers will keep climbing. A few months on, you'll be banging out chin-ups and pull-ups like a pro.

BONUS RESOURCES

- I've created a PDF guide titled, 'How To Become A Chin-Up Champ...And Pull-Up Pro'. It walks you through everything we've just covered, includes picture demonstrations, and would be a handy step-by-step guide to print out. You can download it for free at:

  www.weighttrainingistheway.com/chin-ups

- It's sometimes easier to see all of this in action, so I've created another free video on the Weight Training Is The Way YouTube channel to walk you through mastering chin-ups.

  How To Do Chin-Ups: From Beginner To Pro

  https://www.youtube.com/watch?v=JrA1MLfVo0c

CHAPTER 5

The Trick To Bigger, Stronger Arms

Did you ever hear that story about Arnold Schwarzenegger pretending his biceps were mountains?

Yep, back in his glory days of being a man mountain, The Terminator used to visualise his biceps as being like mountain tops. Arnie claimed his visualisation techniques helped his biceps grow and peak at a massive 22 inches around.

I'm sure you can live without biceps that are bigger than your cranium, but I don't know many guys who don't want bigger, stronger arms.

I even read about a survey Men's Health magazine did a few years ago where 67% of women said they preferred thick arms to a thick penis. We'll just leave it at that.

Now it's obvious why Arnie was doing the whole Austrian mountain visualisation thing: he wanted to develop extra big biceps for flexing in his bodybuilding competitions.

But if you're a bodybuilder then I'm afraid you've picked up the wrong book. I'm really not into all that flexing, posing, fake tan, and super-inflated ego shit.

Instead, my whole weight training ethos has always been helping people become lean, athletic, strong as hell, and developing mental toughness through their gym efforts.

There's never been the need to grow record-breaking biceps that'll be flexed upon a stage while wearing nothing but a smile and budgie-smuggler Speedos.

But, as I said earlier, many guys do get into fitness to develop stronger, more muscular arms. I'm going to explain how you can do exactly that. For women, this same approach will help you sculpt strong, toned arms with good definition.

Now I'm not proclaiming to have arms like Popeye, but they do have good muscle definition, they're strong, and look good in my clothes. Considering they used to resemble twigs before I started lifting weights, I'll take that.

The schoolboy error that most people make when aiming for bigger arms is putting too much emphasis on biceps isolation exercises, such as barbell curls and dumbbell curls.

Thinking of the 'guns' and flexing the head of the bicep, they hit these types of exercise hard. It's the wrong way to go, just ask any experienced weightlifter.

The triceps muscle makes up roughly two thirds of the upper arm, so it naturally makes more sense to put more emphasis on this muscle. It is made up of three heads - long, lateral and medial - and this is why it's known as triceps brachii (Latin for 'three-headed muscle of the arm').

Given that it's the largest muscle in the upper arm, it definitely deserves some special attention. I'll now list my top five exercises for giving your triceps some VIP treatment in the gym...and there's also a video demonstration at the end of the chapter.

Top 5 Triceps Exercises

#1 Dips

Dips is actually a compound exercise because it works several works group at once – triceps, chest, shoulders, forearms and abs. But few exercises work your triceps as effectively as the mighty dips.

The exercise involves holding your body suspended in the air between two parallel bars, lowering your body down until your elbows reach a 90 degree angle, and then pushing back up to the starting position.

Beginners, or people with a lot of weight to lose, can use an assisted machine (just like with chin-ups and pull-ups) at first to develop their strength and increase the number of dips they can perform.

#2 Cable triceps pushdowns

This exercise involves standing upright in front of a cable machine, holding onto a bar at chest level in front of you with your elbows tucked into your side, and then pushing it downwards to engage the triceps.

Straightening your arms downwards and locking out of the elbow works the muscle, but so does the second part where your arms rise back up again in a controlled fashion to the starting position.

A great exercise for isolating the triceps and one where I've seen clients progress quickly in increasing the weight.

#3 Cable triceps pulldowns (reverse of above)

Very similar to the above exercise, except that you're holding the bar with an underhand grip. This also means that you're pulling the bar downwards, rather than pushing.

With your elbows tucked into your side again, and with the underhand grip, this exercise can feel a bit awkward at first. You'll find it's best to lift a bit lighter, compared to the cable triceps pushdown, in order to maintain good technique.

#4 Cable overhead rope extensions

Another cable machine exercise, but this one involves facing away from the machine and using a short rope rather than a bar.

First, set the rope at the top of the pulley. Then, with your heel pressing against the cable machine and holding the rope above your head, step forward with the other leg and lean forward.

Keeping your elbows in position at either side of your head, just like you see in the first picture, extend your arms forward until they're straight out in front of you.

Then bring them back in a controlled fashion, but making sure your elbows stay in the same position at the side of your head. (This will ensure you're working the triceps, rather than bringing your shoulders or back into play).

#5 Narrow grip bench press

Very similar to the bench press, but bringing your arms in closer to slightly narrower than shoulder width. By gripping the bar this way, you put the focus onto your triceps and take your chest muscles largely out of the equation.

A popular move, but not an easy one. Don't make the mistake of thinking you'll be able to lift the same amount of weight as you do in the bench press. It ain't going to happen!

Start lighter with the narrow grip bench press and gradually increase the weight.

The Importance Of Variety To 'Shock' The Muscles Into Development

You must keep mixing it up with the types of exercises you do, the number of sets, and how many repetitions you do each time in the gym. Don't allow your muscles to adapt to the same old routine, you must find fresh ways to keep stressing your muscles in order to force them to grow.

"You've got to shock the muscle, shock the muscle, and shock the muscle with different kinds of training principles." – Arnold Schwarzenegger.

Big Arnie's top triceps moves were: narrow bench press, triceps extensions, and single arm dumbbell triceps extensions (which involves lifting the dumbbell above the head).

Don't Forget...The Mighty Compound Exercises

All of the triceps moves I've described are ridiculously effective for developing the size, strength and muscle definition of your arms.

But it would be daft to get too carried away with triceps isolation exercises on their own in an attempt to grow bigger arms. Compound exercises, such as chin-ups and pull-ups, are devastatingly effective not only for increasing the size of your arms, but for overall upper body development.

I'm forever banging on about the importance of including compound exercises in every weight training workout. I usually recommend a 60/40 or 70/30 percent ratio of compound to isolation exercises, and cover all of my top exercises in my first book in this series, 'Strength Training NOT Bodybuilding' (which is free on Kindle).

If you want to build bigger, stronger arms, while developing good overall body composition, I'd recommend a workout beginning with 4-5 compound exercises, and finishing with 3-4 triceps isolation exercises.

Doing 2-3 sets of each of these exercises will be enough to work the muscles hard enough and stimulate growth, while stripping fat. Below are a couple of workout examples that I've done many times over.

Workout 1:

- Squats x 3 sets (6-9 repetitions each set)
- Bench press x 3 sets (6-9 repetitions each set)
- Chin-ups x 3 sets (6-9 repetitions each set)
- Military press x 3 sets (6-9 repetitions each set)
- Cable triceps pushdown x 3 sets (6-9 repetitions each set)
- Cable triceps pulldown x 3 sets (6-9 repetitions each set)
- Narrow grip bench press x 3 sets (6-9 repetitions each set)

- Dips x 3 sets (Maximum repetitions for each set and then record the total)

Workout 2:

- Deadlifts x 3 sets (6-9 repetitions each set)
- Bent over row x 3 sets (6-9 repetitions each set)
- Upright row x 3 sets (6-9 repetitions each set)
- Clean and press x 3 sets (6-9 repetitions each set)
- Cable overhead rope extension x 3 sets (6-9 repetitions each set)
- Dips x 3 sets (6-9 repetitions each set)
- Cable triceps pushdown x 3 sets (6-9 repetitions each set)

The key here is to put more emphasis on your triceps, rather than your biceps, if you want to develop strong, muscular arms. It's a simple but effective tweak to your workouts, and your biceps will still be worked hard through compound exercises such as: upright row, chin-ups, and bent over row.

A friendly reminder for women: the advice in this chapter does not mean you're going to end up with limbs like The Incredible Hulk. Your much lower testosterone levels won't allow for that. Expect strong, lean, defined arms instead.

BONUS RESOURCES

- I've created another short demonstration video featuring the top five triceps exercises mentioned in this chapter. You can check it out on the Weight Training Is The Way YouTube channel.

- **Weight Training Workout : Best Triceps Exercises** https://www.youtube.com/watch?v=hjc-IzJIUMQ

CHAPTER 6

The Fast Track To Becoming A Lean Machine

How about a workout that strengthens and conditions the entire body?

One that blitzes fat, sculpts rock hard abs, and develops lean muscle at the same time...

And, best of all, one that's done within 15 mins?

You probably thought that kind of workout didn't exist. It does: sprint training. Those two words represent an ultra-effective form of high-intensity exercise that has the potential to completely transform your body shape – and health.

Sprint training triggers a unique, physiological response in the body which, quite literally, turns you into a lean, fat-burning machine.

Remember I covered the positive impact of raising your body's growth hormone levels earlier? Well, sprint training supercharges your body's natural production of growth hormone, with some studies showing that levels more than QUADRUPLE and stay elevated for longer.

Those are the many upsides of pretending you're an Olympic sprinter for 15 minutes. Here's the downside: it's excruciatingly difficult.

I'm talking: heart pounding like it's going to smash through your ribcage, legs shaking like Elvis on 10 pints of Red Bull, and breathlessness like you've just smoked every cigarette on a whirlwind tour of the Marlboro factory.

But don't worry, that's just your first session. It gets better...slightly.

While the intense nature of sprinting like a maniac for 15 mins is tough as hell, the benefits are huge and make every second of the serious grind worth it.

I've been hooked on weight training and the world of fitness for a long while now, and it still surprises me how little exposure sprint training receives. Considering the massive benefits, I don't hear enough about it, or see enough people pulling on their running trainers and getting stuck into it.

I'll delve into the benefits you need to know about later in this chapter, and I'll lay out a simple plan for executing on an effective 15 mins sprinting session, no matter what level of fitness you're at.

But first, I want you to think back to a time when you watched the Olympics or Commonwealth Games on TV? The 100 metres sprint was usually the most exciting event, right?

The tension in the air as the athletes loosened up before being told to take their spot on the track. Their legs rising and back arching in anticipation after the words "on your marks" echoed round the silent stadium. A row of muscular legs and arms bursting out of the traps after the gun is fired.

And then...a short, intense, electric 10 secs of action where one hundredth of a second makes all the difference between silver and gold.

Now I want you think about that time you saw a 100 metres sprint athlete that had an average looking physique.

That's right, you didn't! Every one of the sprint athletes – the men and women – have bodies like Greek Gods. Strong, muscular arms, rounded shoulders and chest, clearly-defined abs, and powerful thighs.

And to get to that level, they had clearly built mental strength to match their incredible physiques.

If you watched the 100 metres sprint, there's a chance you might also have tuned into the 10,000 metres race.

They're another group of athletes aiming to complete the distance in the fastest time, yet they generally have thinner bodies with much less muscle mass.

Both groups are runners, and both are athletes competing at the highest level, so what's the difference?

Once again, it largely comes down to hormones. The short, sharp intense bursts of speed with sprint training triggers the release of high amounts of growth hormone. This not only burns fat, but develops muscle tissue too.

Long distance running, on the other hand, simply doesn't have the same physiological effect. While growth hormone levels are lower, the calorie demand is higher for the prolonged period of exercise.

This form of training will eat into muscle after glycogen and fat stores run low.

Let's sprint head first into the whys of sprint training, then we'll run over exactly how to do it.

7 Reasons To Sprint Faster Than Forrest Gump

#1 Anti-aging effect and immune system boost

This is all down to the anabolic hormone effect. Growth hormone is known for stimulating growth, cell regeneration and reproduction. Growth hormone also plays various other roles in the body including enhancing the immune system.

As described in the chapter on Tabata protocol, high-intensity interval training can trigger the creation of new mitochondria in your cells; slowing the aging process.

#2 Extreme fat burning

Sprinting really revs up your metabolism and continues to strip fat long after your workout has ended. In fact, a study carried out in 2013 showed that sprints increased fat oxidation by 75%.

Ten healthy men, aged in their 20s, took part in the study and were involved in four 30 second bouts of cycle sprints, with little rest in between, followed by almost five minutes of rest at the end.

The huge fat burning rate was recorded, while blood pressure levels were also shown to be reduced afterwards.

#3 It produces other muscle-building hormones

Sprinting stimulates the production of other anabolic hormones that are key to the muscle building process, including testosterone and IGF1.

The results of a study published in The Journal of Strength And Conditioning Research in August 2011 demonstrated this.

The research involved 12 young men and showed that levels of testosterone and IGF1, along with growth hormone, were all elevated after various 100m-400m sprints.

#4 Your sprinting session only takes 15-20 mins

As sprint training involves short, sharp bursts of speed over distances of around 60m-100m, followed by quick rest periods, the entire session can be done in as little as 15 mins.

It's an ideal form of exercise for people who are short on time – and short on cash. You obviously don't need a gym membership for sprint training or any fancy equipment. Just head to a local park, ideally with a slight hill, and get into action.

Remember it's best to train in the morning on an empty stomach for maximum effect.

#5 It strengthens the heart

Regular exercise is recommended for people with high blood pressure, and it appears that high-intensity training is more effective than moderate exercise for improving the situation.

Comparing 30 minutes of moderate exercise to several bouts of high-intensity training (HIT), lasting 1-4 minutes, researchers concluded that HIT is "superior to CMT (continuous moderate training) for improving cardiorespiratory fitness".

Their findings published in the American Journal of Cardiovascular Disease in 2012 also showed that intense exercise was shown to have positive effects on arterial stiffness and insulin sensitivity.

#6 It strengthens the mind

We all know how exercise is good for your mental health. But there's nothing like pushing yourself to the absolute max physically to build self-esteem, strength, character and confidence.

Just as former Navy Seal David Goggins – known as the "toughest man alive" – puts it: "The true benefit of working out for me is what it does to your mindset. While looking better is always a great added plus, the animalistic mentality that comes with getting after it on the regular is truly where I benefitted the most. It's the repetition and self-discipline that changes the self-esteem from the inside out."

If you do sprint training properly – and I mean running flat-out at your maximum effort – you'll find that you muster up mental toughness just to get through a session. The mind will come up with all sorts of excuses to quit, slow down, or do one sprint less than your target.

By pushing through and sticking with your goals, your confidence will grow along with your fitness levels. You'll also develop discipline and mental strength that'll help you achieve positive results in other areas of your life.

#7 It sculpts six pack abs

Sprint training is a very explosive form of exercise, first engaging the glutes, hamstrings, calves and shoulders as you launch from the starting point.

The movement of your hips and arms as your thrust forward step by step also work your abdominal muscles hard, particularly the obliques at either side of your stomach.

This motion, coupled with the rush of anabolic hormones, strips away stubborn fat from around the waist. The main reason most people have never seen their abdominal muscles is because they simply have a layer of fat covering them.

You could do countless crunches, sit-ups, or strap one of those expensive electrical six pack belts round your waist. But unless your bodyfat levels are reduced, your abs will never show.

Sprint training is one of the best ways to lose flab around your belly and finally see some muscle shape and definition there.

Go From Running Rookie To Sprints Superhero

Sprint training, done properly, is damn hard. No point in me sugar-coating it. But I'm sure you've heard the very true statement, "nothing worth having comes easy."

Same goes for your fitness, physique, health, and the rock-solid mindset we all want. That's why you should embrace the toughness of sprint training and just dive deep into them.

There are levels to this and, like anything, you can progress up them with repetition and dedication. Here's how to get started and move through the different phases as you gradually improve your sprinting performance and overall fitness.

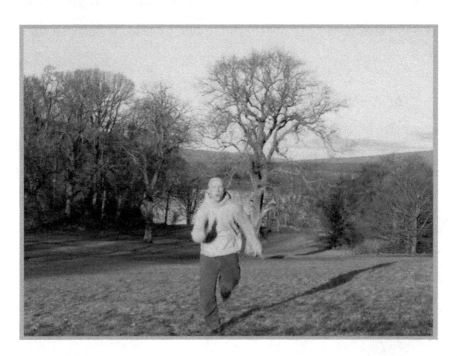

BEGINNER

Distance: 50-60 yards.

Sprints: 5-6.

- Step 1: Head outdoors to somewhere like a local park, and find a stretch of flat ground that's not very busy with people.
- Step 2: Set a start and finish point, with a distance of around 50-60 yards between them.
- Step 3: Warm up well for several minutes by doing a light jog, stretches for your arms and legs (particularly the hamstrings), star jumps, bodyweight squats etc.
- Step 4: Ready for launch...and sprint as fast as possible to your marker point.
- Step 5: Walk back to where you started, breathing in deep through your nose to get plenty of oxygen back in your system. Focus on all the benefits your sprinting efforts will bring, not giving any room in your mind for excuses.
- Step 6: Once you get to the starting point, turn and set off again, running flat out at full speed. Repeat the process for 5-6 sprints.

INTERMEDIATE

Distance: 100 yards.

Sprints: 7-8.

- Step 1: Head outdoors to somewhere like a local park, and find a stretch of flat ground or a hill with a slight incline.
- Step 2: Set a start and finishing point, with a distance of around 100 yards between them.
- Step 3: Warm up properly for several minutes before you begin. A light jog and leg and arm stretches will do the trick.
- Step 4: Set off and sprint as fast as you can to your finish line marker point.
- Step 5: Walk back to the starting point, breathing deeply to recover as much as you can and stay fully focused on the amazing results sprint training brings.
- Step 6: As soon as you reach the starting point, sprint again at maximum effort till you reach your marker. Repeat for 7-8 sprints.

ELITE ATHLETE

Distance: 120-150 yards.

Sprints: 9-12.

- Step 1: Find a hill in a park, or a quiet road with an incline that's not too steep.
- Step 2: Set a start and finishing point, with a distance of around 120 yards between them.

- Step 3: Make sure you warm up properly for several minutes, with several and leg and arm stretches, along with a light jog.
- Step 4: Set off and sprint as fast as you can to your finish line marker point.
- Step 5: Walk back to the starting point, breathe deep and focus on all the benefits your sprinting efforts will bring, not giving any room for excuses.
- Step 6: As soon as you reach the starting point, sprint again at maximum effort till you reach your marker. Repeat for 9-12 sprints.

BONUS RESOURCES

I've created a short demo video to complement this chapter and help motivate you into getting started with sprint training. Check it out on the YouTube channel.

Sprint Training For Building Muscle And Fat Loss:
https://www.youtube.com/watch?v=FlPePUVGBgl

CHAPTER 7

Negative Training For Some Seriously Positive Results

What would you say if I told you that you only had to do 1.5 repetitions of each exercise in the gym to build some serious muscle?

What if I told you those 1.5 repetitions would also incinerate fat?

I'm guessing the response would go something like: "Stop talking bullshit. Right now. You clown."

You'd maybe even consider not reading another word of this book if you thought I was being serious.

I am being serious...but stick with me on this. Keep reading!

When I say 1.5 repetitions, I don't mean any old repetition. I'm talking monster reps. I'm talking 1.5 feels like 1.5 thousand reps first time around.

I'm referring to what's known as 'negative accentuated training', a unique way of working out with dumbbells, barbells and resistance machines in the gym that has been proven to deliver amazing results.

It's not widely known or followed in the fitness industry, but science has shown that negative training can help men and women achieve rapid fat loss, while gaining several pounds of muscle, in a matter of weeks.

I'll give some examples later and I'll properly explain all the ins and outs of negative accentuated training. I'll also show how you can incorporate this new style of exercise into your gym workout programme and take your strength to new levels.

Firstly, I'll briefly cover what I consider to be the most effective and efficient way to exercise to build a lean, strong, athletic body, while also maintaining optimal physical and mental health.

1) Lift heavy weights three times per week, one day on and one day off.
2) Throw in an additional high-intensity training session each week (i.e. sprint training).
3) Ensure that compound exercises make up at least 50% of your weights workouts.
4) Increase the load as you get stronger, always pushing for personal bests.
5) Mix up your workout programme to keep things exciting and challenge yourself.

That's it in five simple steps. As for the types of exercises, how much weight you should lift, and the different training systems I've been using for the past 20 years in my gym programmes, there's no point in me going over all of that again here.

It's all covered in my first book *Strength Training NOT Bodybuilding: Build Muscle & Lose Fat...Without Morphing Into A Bodybuilder - https://www.amazon.com/dp/B0774G2ZL8*, which is free to download on Kindle.

What I'll re-iterate is the importance of variety in your gym programme and switching things up. No consecutive workouts should be the same in any given week. No single training system should be used throughout a 10-12 week programme.

Otherwise, the body quickly adapts and muscle growth and development is limited. It'll also result in your training hitting a plateau and a slower rate of fat loss.

For example, I used to run a 10-week online training programme, which would be set up as follows:

Weeks 1-2: Mainly compound exercises, using the 'triple heavy' training system.

Weeks 3-5: Introducing more muscle isolation exercises, switch to the 'three set shocker' training system.

Weeks 6-7: Bring in more new exercises, switch to the 'drop sets' training system, and introduce a 'finisher' exercise.

Weeks 8-10: Continue mixing up order of exercises, switch to the 'slow burner' training system.

I've sworn by switching things up this way for the best part of 20 years, and those four training systems I mentioned have been at the centre of my weights workouts.

In the past few months I've recently added a fifth – negative accentuated training. It's been one of the best - and worst - things I've done for my training.

Best...because it takes strength training to a deeper level, hitting muscle fibres that don't usually get hit, and triggering fresh growth and development.

Worst...because my first couple of sessions were torture. I wasn't just taken out of my comfort zone, it was like I was brutally abducted.

Introducing...Negative Accentuated Training

The standard advice in the fitness industry for muscle growth and development is 'progressive overload', which basically means gradually increasing the weight in your exercises as you get stronger.

The negative accentuated method is different in three aspects: the amount of weight lifted, the duration of each rep, and an emphasis being placed on the eccentric part of the exercise.

Each exercise in your gym workouts include an 'eccentric' part of the movement and 'concentric'; which are also referred to as negative and positive.

The lifting/raising part of the repetition = concentric/positive.

The lowering part of the repetition = eccentric/negative.

For example, you begin doing barbell curls with the bar resting against your thighs and then curl the bar up towards your chest. This motion of lifting the bar is concentric and squeezing your muscles shortens the biceps muscles it's targeting.

The second part of the exercise involves lowering the bar in a controlled manner to the starting position, which is eccentric and lengthens the biceps muscles again.

Typically, each part of the movement takes just a couple of seconds to complete. Up for 2 secs and down for 2, or maybe 3, secs.

The difference with negative accentuated training is that each movement is much slower and takes 30 secs to complete – and there's an additional negative part thrown in for good measure.

It's no longer: positive (lifting) for 2 secs > negative (lowering) for 2 secs.

Instead, we do: negative (lowering) for 30 secs > positive (lifting) for 30 secs > negative again for another 30 secs.

Sound simple enough? It's not, trust me.

The 'slow burner' training system I've used for years is similar in that the negative part of the exercise is extended, but that's only for 5 secs and comes nowhere near the intensity of 30 secs negative > 30 secs positive > followed by 30 secs negative again.

I'm fairly new to this tough training system, having only introduced it into my own gym programme about four months ago. Therefore, while I've seen noticeable strength and muscle gain through negative accentuated training, I'm not claiming to be an expert on it.

Dr Ellington Darden PhD, one of the world's leading authorities on weight training and sports nutrition, is the main man when it comes to negative accentuated training.

He has written dozens of fitness books and it was his 2014 book *'Body Fat Breakthrough: Tap The Muscle-Building Power Of Negative Training And Lose Up To 30 Pounds in 30 Days' - http://https/www.amazon.com/dp/1623361036/* that convinced me to give this new training method a try.

It's an area of training he's spent decades researching and refining, and what impresses me most about Dr Darden's work is the evidence he gathers. Not only does he give recommendations based on scientific research, he also sets up his own studies to measure the effectiveness of what he preaches.

In 2012, Dr Darden did a study in Gainesville, USA, involving 40 women and 25 men. All were put on a fat loss diet and exercise plan, which consisted of restricted calories each day, drinking a gallon of cold water each day, and doing two days of negative accentuated exercises in the gym.

The results after just six weeks were pretty astounding. The men, average of 48, lost an average of 29lbs and gained almost 9lbs of muscle. The women, at an average age of 43, lost almost 17lbs of fat and gained just over 5lbs of muscle.

While the results of these people are very impressive, they shouldn't be too surprising considering the benefits of negative accentuated training.

Science has shown that it involves more muscle fibres than standard weightlifting; notably additional fast-twitch muscle fibres – which contribute mainly to muscle growth. It also causes more tiny muscle fibre tears, which sparks the muscle-building process.

It also works the entire joint structure, leading to more strength. The unique method of working out with 1.5 reps also allows for more work in less time, helping you train more efficiently.

How You Can Implement Negative Accentuated Training

When doing negative accentuated training, Dr Darden recommends lifting around 80% of the weight you would normally pump out for 8-12 repetitions. That should be the aim, but it's extremely difficult.

I'm experienced in lifting weights and I couldn't manage 80% for the full 90 secs training duration on ANY of my exercises at first. This method of training was a shock to the system, and so I began at around 60% for the first few sessions – and worked my way up to 80% in subsequent workouts.

Your repetitions can be between 20 and 30 secs, therefore you have the option to adjust both the time and weight in your workouts week by week.

Let's say it's time to change things up with your weights workouts and you decide to use the negative accentuated training system for the next four weeks in the gym.

Here's an example of how you could implement it into your workouts:

STANDARD WORKOUT - 3 sets of every exercise with usual technique and increasing the weight if you complete 9 or more repetitions.

Bench press – 70kg/155lbs

Military press – 40kg/90lbs

Lat pulldown – 50kg/110lbs

Dips – maximum reps over 3 sets.

Dumbbell flyes – 20kg/45lbs

Cable triceps pushdown – 40kg/90lbs

Overhead rope extension – 30kg/65lbs

NEGATIVE ACCENTUATED WORKOUT - 2 sets of every exercise and increasing the weight for the second set if you complete the <u>full</u> exercise duration.

Bench press – 40kg/90lbs (20 secs lowering bar > 20 secs pushing bar > 20 secs lowering bar).

Military press – 25kg/55lbs (20 secs lowering bar > 20 secs pushing bar > 20 secs lowering bar).

Lat pulldown – 30kg/65lbs (20 secs raising bar > 20 secs pulling bar > 20 secs raising bar).

Assisted machine dips – set pin to 30kg/65lbs for support (20 secs lowering body > 20 secs pushing upwards > 20 secs lowering body).

Dumbbell flyes – 12.5kg/27.5lbs (20 secs lowering dumbbells > 20 secs raising dumbbells > 20 secs lowering).

Cable triceps pushdown – 25kg/55lbs (20 secs raising bar > 20 secs pushing bar downwards > 20 secs raising bar).

Overhead rope extension – 20kg/45lbs (20 secs releasing rope backwards from front extension > 20 secs pulling rope forward > 20 secs releasing rope backwards).

As you can see, the weights level for each exercise has been reduced by around 60% compared to the previously described standard workout. (Remember, these are just weight load examples...not an expectation of what you should be lifting).

After three of these negative accentuated sessions in one week, you'll be feeling stronger and more confident. This is when you can start increasing the weight and/or time duration to make more progress.

Here's how your negative accentuated training plan could look:

Week 1

- Two sets of 7 exercises.
- Around 60% of usual weight.
- 20 secs negative > 20 secs positive > 20 secs negative for each exercise.

Week 2

- Two sets of 8 exercises.
- Around 70% of usual weight.
- 20 secs negative > 20 secs positive > 20 secs negative for each exercise.

Week 3

- Two sets of 8 exercises.
- Around 70% of usual weight.
- 25 secs negative > 25 secs positive > 25 secs negative.

Week 4

- Two sets of 8 exercises.
- Around 70% of usual weight.
- 30 secs negative > 30 secs positive > 30 secs negative.

This approach will definitely help you adjust to this difficult, but very effective form of training.

BONUS RESOURCES

- To help you get to grips with negative accentuated training, I've created a short video on the Weight Training Is The Way Youtube channel. Enjoy!
- **Negative Training For More Muscle...And Less Fat:** https://www.youtube.com/watch?v=YfrCXqiApc4

NUTRITION HACKS

CHAPTER 8

Superfoods That Fight Inflammation

"Inflammation is at the root of nearly all disease."

I remember being pretty shocked when I first read those words about 10 years ago. My throat was red raw with yet another bout of tonsillitis and I'd decided to do some research to try to figure out what the hell was going on.

After an extended hunt on the Kindle store on Amazon, it led me to a book about inflammation and how chronic inflammation in our tissues and organs is at the centre of virtually all our ills.

To quickly sum up in the simplest fashion: our bodies have an inflammatory response to injury/bacteria/food/toxins/stress in everyday life. It's designed to heal the body, and the obvious signs are heat, redness, pain and swelling.

A healthy person who handles this process of acute inflammation can restore balance in hours or a couple of days. But the problems occur when inflammation is prolonged.

When inflammation burns too much for too long, the body breaks down and disease spreads. This is known as 'chronic inflammation'. You could say our insides are on fire!

The bottom line is: if you want to be healthy, strong and perform at your best in and out of the gym then doing what you can to reduce inflammation is a very important step.

Reducing inflammation to lower levels is key to the optimal functioning of your body, your immune system, for having more energy, mental clarity, and simply feeling more vibrant.

This point is particularly pertinent to people who exercise several times per week because intense training causes inflammation in the joints and muscles.

You know what I mean - that can-barely-walk-sore-thighs feeling you get a day or two after doing squats in the gym. Or the stiff shoulders you get the morning after doing push-ups for the first time in months.

Proper rest and recovery is crucial for cooling your inflamed muscles and joints after tough workouts, and that's why I always recommend a day's rest in between weightlifting sessions or high-intensity training. I'll cover that in more detail in a later chapter.

But nutrition also plays a hugely important role. Specific foods are known to be fantastic firefighters when it comes to inflammation and it's beneficial to include more of them in your diet.

I'll cover the best ones in this chapter, while in the next chapter I'll highlight problem foods which are notorious for causing an inflammatory response in our bodies. Some may surprise you, but if you avoid/limit them you can potentially see big improvements in your health and wellbeing, as well as faster recovery from your workouts.

All Natural Foods That Help Beat Inflammation

Spices in particular have strong anti-inflammatory properties, however some vegetables like dark-coloured greens and broccoli are effective too. Foods high in omega 3 fatty acids including fish, egg yolks, and grass-fed meats are also good anti-inflammatory food sources.

Below I've listed the most potent foods proven to reduce inflammation in the body, and even if they're not part of your diet right now, it's very easy to introduce them into main meal recipes and shakes.

Turmeric

This super spice has been used in Ayurvedic and Chinese medicine for centuries due to its potent anti-inflammatory, anti-fungal, antioxidant, and anti-viral properties. Several good reasons to eat more curry!

Health experts point to the 'curcumin' antioxidant within turmeric that dramatically reduces inflammation, improves insulin resistance, and even fights the growth of tumour cells in various cancers.

However, its bioavailability is low when consumed on its own. This is increased big time when taken with black pepper, and some clever chap came up with the idea of pairing turmeric and pepper together in supplemental capsule form. You can also buy these pretty cheaply online via Amazon.

Turmeric also contains more than 20 other anti-inflammatory compounds, including six COX-2 inhibitors (COX-2 is an enzyme which speeds up inflammation and pain).

Of course you can add more turmeric to your diet by an extra dash or two more in home-made curry recipes, or you can add it to meat or fish marinades. There are also some turmeric-infused teas available, but I nearly choked on the first (and last ever) one I drank.

Ginger

Ginger is one of the healthiest – and tastiest spices – on earth. It is packed with nutrients and compounds that have a positive affect on your body and brain.

Gingerol is the main bioactive compound within the spice that has powerful anti-inflammatory and antioxidant effects. Antioxidants get rid of free radicals in our system that damage cells – and lead to inflammation.

These are the main reasons ginger has long been used in different forms of traditional and alternative medicine.

Ginger has been found to be effective in improving digestion, fighting the flu and common cold, as well as reducing nausea. It has even been shown to help with muscle pain and soreness, which is not surprising considering how it cools inflammation.

A study was carried out in 2010 to show the effects ginger had on relieving muscle pain caused by exercise. One group of 34 people consumed 2g of raw ginger for 11 consecutive days, while another group of 40 people had 2g of heated ginger over the same period.

They performed 18 different arm exercises to induce inflammation and muscle soreness afterwards.

Various markers were analysed before and three days after exercise, and researchers found that raw ginger reduced muscle pain by 25% a day after exercise compared to placebo, while the heated ginger brought pain down by 23%.

Researchers concluded: "This study demonstrates that daily consumption of raw and heat-treated ginger resulted in moderate-to-large reductions in muscle pain following exercise-induced muscle injury.

"Our findings agree with those showing hypoalgesic effects of ginger in osteoarthritis patients and further demonstrate ginger's effectiveness as a pain reliever."

You can easily introduce ginger to your diet by adding ½ tsp of ground ginger to your protein shake/healthy smoothie. It's a key ingredients in many of the shake recipes in my book _Meal Prep: 50 Simple Recipes For Health & Fitness Nuts_ – _https://www.amazon.com/dp/B072J1SMCZ_.

Cinnamon

Cinnamon is another really tasty spice that has strong anti-inflammatory properties. It's also known for stabilising blood sugar levels, as well as containing antibacterial and antioxidant compounds.

It's an all-round super spice for balance and wellness, but make sure you buy the right stuff though as there are two major types available – 'ceylon' or 'cassia' cinnamon.

Ceylon is the real deal, produced by the ceylon tree native to Sri Lanka, and is much better for your body. You can buy organic ceylon cinnamon online via Amazon.

A study published in 2015 which highlighted the positive effects certain bio-active compounds in cinnamon had on inflammation.

Researchers concluded: "If therapeutic concentrations can be achieved in target tissues, cinnamon and its components may be useful in the treatment of age-related inflammatory conditions."

It's also easy to include cinnamon in your diet in your breakfast oats, shakes/healthy smoothies, yoghurts etc.

Cayenne pepper

Another spice used as a medicine for millennia by Native Americans, and also used as an alternative treatment in countries across Asia for many years for digestive and circulation problems.

It contains various antioxidants that mop up free radicals, protecting against cellular damage that leads to inflammation and disease in the longer term.

The compound capsaicin gives cayenne pepper its spicy kick – and is also responsible for its medicinal properties. Capsaicin depletes nerve cells of substance P, which is a chemical that sends pain signals to the brain.

It's simple to introduce more cayenne pepper into your diet through tasty chilli, chicken or even soup recipes.

Cloves

It's less likely that this spice will be part of your everyday diet, cloves seem to make more of an appearance in the winter time, being used in mulled wine and ground down to be added to mixtures for stewing meats etc.

But it's so potent that it's worth sharing its benefits with you here. Cloves contain eugenol, similar to cinnamon's cinnamaldehye (xix), but even more powerful. Eugenol blocks the COX-2 enzyme that causes inflammation, and also provides fibre, manganese, vitamin K and vitamin C.

Cloves are also antifungal and have antimicrobial properties, killing off three common strains of bacteria including E-coli.

Oily fish

I always remember my mum having cod liver oil capsules in the house when I was a kid. The thought of swallowing the oil from the liver of a fish made me screw my face up whenever I saw them in the kitchen cupboard.

Turns out my mum is smarter than I give her credit for, because this food supplement is high in omega-3 fatty acids and is also loaded with vitamins A and D.

Omega-3 fatty acids in food help reduce inflammation throughout the body, and some studies have shown added benefits for heart health, brain function and people with diabetes.

They also balance blood sugar and build all cell membranes in the body. Every message your cells need to survive is communicated through cell membranes, therefore having sufficient supplies of omega-3 in your diet to help them function properly is vital.

Mackerel is the richest source of omega 3 (5,134mg per 100g/3.5oz serving), salmon is next (2,260mg per 100g serving), while one tablespoon of cod liver oil (spewing at the thought) provides 2,664mg of omega 3.

Herring (1,729mg per 100g serving) and sardines (1,480mg per 100g serving) also pack a decent omega 3 punch.

Omega 3 is a family of fats, including ALA, EPA and DHA, however ALA (alpha-linolenic-acid) cannot be made by the body so we must get this from our diet.

The UK Association of Dietitians recommends that everyone should try to eat two portions of fish per week, one of which should be oily fish.

Don't like fish? You can also get omega-3 from nuts, seeds and leafy green vegetables. Below are some other good sources.

Flaxseed/Linseed

These small brown or yellow seeds are the richest whole foods source of the omega-3 fat ALA. They're often milled or used to make flaxseed oil, which is a popular health supplement.

Along with its high omega-3 content (2,338mg per tablespoon of whole seeds), flaxseeds are also very high in fibre, magnesium, vitamin E and several other nutrients.

What I love most about flaxseed/linseed is that it's so easy to include in your diet. Sprinkle milled flaxseed/linseed over oats, cereal, or blend it up in your protein shakes/healthy smoothies.

I have 2-3 tablespoons of milled linseed (£2 pouch from Aldi) in my daily superfood shake, which also includes protein powder, frozen fruits, cinnamon or ginger, coconut milk etc. These shakes are packed with inflammation-fighting ingredients – and taste amazing.

Chia seeds

Okay, I know what you're thinking: "who the hell actually eats Chia seeds?"

I'll be honest, I rarely have them myself. But they are absolutely another rich source of those inflammation-fighting omega-3s. One ounce/28g of these tiny seeds pack an impressive 4,952mg of omega-3.

So it might well be worth picking them up next time you're in the supermarket or health food store. Just like flaxseed, you can simply throw a tablespoon of these into your blender while whizzing up a healthy smoothie.

Walnuts

At 2,542mg of omega-3 in every ounce serving (or about seven walnuts), these bad boys can also help keep inflammation in check. Walnuts are also good sources of antioxidants, fibre, and contain high amounts of copper, manganese, and vitamin E.

Walnuts and almonds are a great healthy snack alternative to chocolate, sweets and crisps. They are a good plant-based source of protein and healthy fats.

It might be time to add a few more items onto your weekly shopping list. Now let's look at some items you might want to remove, or at least limit in your diet. Your body will thank you for it.

CHAPTER 9

Inflammatory Foods To Avoid...And Healthier Alternatives

Don't believe anyone who tries to sell you onto the perfect diet...because there simply isn't one.

To your average Joe and Josephine Bloggs, diet is split into two camps: healthy foods and unhealthy foods. Now I'm a fan of simplifying diet and nutrition as much as possible, but it's a little trickier than that.

We humans are a special breed and, while one food might be healthy and nutritious for you, that very same food could hurt your mum, or your next-door neighbour. By 'hurt' I'm talking stomach cramps, indigestion, diarrhoea, a sore throat...all common symptoms when people have an inflammatory response to food or drink.

This is all down to food sensitivities and intolerances. While most people can eat most foods without any real issues, the fact is that some items in our diet cause flare-ups in our system, and some problem foods can cause outright chaos.

Where I live in the UK, it's estimated that around 45% of the population are suffering from food intolerances, according to Allergy UK. This is no huge surprise in our Western society where ready meals, takeaways and sugar-laden processed junk are the norm.

Eating these types of foods regularly robs our body of nutrients, hampers our immune system function, messes up our gut microbiome, and creates an acidic environment in our bodies; all of which goes hand in hand with inflammation.

And remember, chronic inflammation is at the root of most disease. I realise I'm probably sounding like the Grim Reaper on a bad day right now, but it gets better, I promise.

After highlighting inflammatory foods worth cutting out – or at least reducing in your diet - I'll then serve up some awesome alternatives that are healthy, tasty, and won't set your insides on fire.

It'd be impossible for me to tell you right now what foods, if any, don't agree with you. Although I'd guess there are some you already avoid because they upset your guts. As I mentioned already, our bodies are all different and people don't always respond the same to certain foods.

What complicates matters even more is that you may well have food sensitivities you simply didn't realise. It's well known that eating a single peanut can be fatal for some people as it can cause such an extreme, anaphylactic reaction.

This is a food allergy and in some other cases we see other strong reactions such as swelling of the face and tongue, eczema or hives.

But we can also have a lower grade inflammatory response to other foods and drinks, which don't cause serious issues but can affect your immune system and overall health over time.

I'm not here to preach one diet over the other, or demonise foods that some people love and have been enjoying for years. Instead, what I'm going to do is simply highlight a select group of 'common inflammatory foods'; the ones that researchers suggest are the fire-starters in the bodies of some people.

Then it's over to you. You can do more research, make changes to your diet, or do nothing at all. This book is all about fitness and nutrition hacks, and simply removing some of these inflammatory foods may well be the most important hack you implement.

I strongly believe that what we exclude from our diets is just as important for our health, wellbeing and performance as what we include.

Common Food Intolerances That Trigger Inflammation

Gluten (wheat, barley, rye, oats)

Gluten is a family of proteins found in grains including wheat, barley, rye, oats and spelt. 'Glu-ten' is added to many of our foods to act like a glue, helping the likes of bread to rise and keep its shape.

Problem is, this glue-like protein is not easily broken down by some people and can cause digestive distress and inflammation elsewhere in the body.

Gluten intolerance does not just affect people with celiac disease or other serious bowel disorders, and awareness of the problems this protein causes for some people is becoming more widespread.

It has been estimated that milder forms of gluten sensitivity affect up to one third of all Americans. Bloating, constipation, diarrhoea, headaches and stomach pains are just some of the symptoms associated with gluten intolerance.

The gluten in common foods like bread, oats, pasta, and cereal trigger an inflammatory response and the symptoms I've just described are the warning signs from the body that all is not well.

The wider medical community still largely ignores the effects food allergies and sensitivities have on our health, however research in the prestigious journal 'Science' and the journal 'Gut' has confirmed the direct link between what we eat and how we feel.

"Dealing with food allergies is essential to creating wellness of mind, body and brain."

- *Dr Mark Hyman, author of The Ultra Mind Solution.*

Of all the gluten-containing grains, wheat is the most commonly consumed. Simply removing that from the diet can help people with gut issues or other noticeable symptoms following eating.

Dairy (milk, cheese, butter, yoghurt)

Did you used to guzzle gallons of milk when you were a kid? Drink a pint in one go straight from the carton? Drive your mum nuts as there was barely enough milk left for a cup of tea?

I was in that mad-for-milk club too. We know that milk is nutritious for kids and is a good source of calcium for developing stronger teeth and bones.

What's not so well known is that when we get older, many people cannot properly digest milk.

There are two reasons for this: because of a sugar it contains called lactose, or because of a protein called casein A1.

It's been estimated that two thirds of people across the globe have a reduced ability to digest lactose after infancy, according to the National Institutes of Health (NIH). Your genetics has a lot to do with whether or not you end up lactose intolerant.

Symptoms of lactose intolerance usually appear within a few hours of consuming milk or other dairy products containing lactose, and these include: farting, diarrhoea, a bloated stomach, cramps, headaches, and feeling sick.

Some people can drinking a glass of milk symptom free, while others may not even be able to have a splash of milk in their coffee.

Lactose intolerance is a widespread issue, but casein A1 protein is a lesser-known but bigger problem. Around half a century ago, the cows in Northern Europe went through a genetic mutation due to changes in farming and their diet.

Their milk became full of the casein A1 protein, which is transformed into another protein called beta-casomorphin when drank. The problem is that beta-casomorphin can trigger an immune reaction and make you feel sick.

While it's estimated that two thirds of people are lactose intolerant, the symptoms of many people may actually be caused by A1 intolerance.

Either way, there's healthy alternatives on the market these days which are much easier to digest and healthier. I'll cover them at the end of this chapter.

Eggs

Eggs are very nutritious, packed with vitamins, and are one of the world's most-eaten superfoods. However, some people have an egg intolerance, which is often only to the egg white.

Some of the symptoms that occur include bloating, heartburn, headaches, and an upset stomach. Prevention is simply by avoiding/limiting eggs in your diet, and foods that contain eggs, such as mayonnaise or cakes and cookies.

Peanuts

Peanuts are "one of the worst ingredients for your health", according to Dr Steven Gundry, author of The Plant Paradox. Although a good source of protein, peanuts are also jam-packed with lectins, which can also cause digestive distress and inflammation in some people.

The gluten mentioned earlier is actually a form of lectin. Gluten is not the only bad guy, according to Dr Gundry and other health experts, such as Joe Cohen, of Selfhacked.com. They insist that foods containing high levels of lectins should be avoided big time.

The lectins topic is a whole other book on its own, but suffice to say that the small peanut is the worst offender, and you can easily replace it with other healthier nuts and nut butters.

How To Identify And Remove Problem Foods

I want to stress two important things once again:

#1 I'm not demonising food and suggesting you remove some, or any, of the above items.

#2 Food sensitivities/intolerances don't affect everyone.

But the fact is that some foods that are healthy for some people may cause health issues for others. An inflammatory response, day after day, just through eating can affect your health, wellbeing, and performance in and out of the gym.

The best way to discover if you have gluten or other food sensitivities is to try an elimination diet, removing suspected problem foods for 2-3 weeks and gauging how you feel during that time. It may be that headaches ease up, phleghm in your throat disappears, or your stomach becomes less bloated.

There are also various options online for food sensitivity tests where you post blood samples and lab tests are done against various foods and ingredients; more than 200 in some cases.

Healthy Alternatives To Stock Up On

Whether you suspect you have intolerances or not, there are still simple steps you can take immediately to remove those most common inflammatory foods.

Don't worry, you're life is not over if you quit peanut butter or your usual cow's milk. There are excellent alternatives available, some of which I've listed below.

A2 milk, or goat's milk

There are still plenty of cows roaming around Southern Europe that never went through the genetic mutation. They produce a different type of protein, casein A2, in their milk which is much easier to digest and doesn't cause the same inflammatory response.

Goat's milk is also a great option and is considered nutritionally superior to cow's milk. It's high in many essential nutrients, and is a good source of vitamins and minerals such as calcium and riboflavin.

Non-dairy milk

There are various dairy-free types on milk in most supermarkets nowadays. Rice milk, almond, cashew milk, oat milk etc.

I personally find most of them pretty tasteless and watery, apart from cashew milk, which I'd say is the best of the bunch.

Grass-fed French or Italian butter

The cows in Southern France and Italy don't produce casein A1, therefore they produce casein A2 butter that's much healthier for you.

As well as being easier to digest, this type of butter tastes even better. It's richer and creamier, and you'll probably not want to eat another type of butter again.

Goat's yoghurt

Some anti-inflammatory compounds are found in goat's milk. One of those is oligosaccharides, also known as short-chain sugar molecules, which make it easier for humans to digest milk.

When fermented, goat's milk also makes a tasty yoghurt filled with good bacteria that improves digestive health and functioning. Because of this, I have a small amount of goat's yoghurt every couple of days.

Almond butter (instead of peanut butter)

Listen, I love peanut butter as much as you. It was like a death in the family saying goodbye to that crunchy, spreadable goodness.

But when you introduce almond butter into your kitchen instead, life becomes complete again.

Even better, my local health food store do almond butter with coconut. It's the best thing since sliced bread and almond butter with coconut.

Gluten free foods

You can find gluten-free options on most restaurant menus nowadays, and there is a 'free from' section in most supermarkets where you can pick up bread, wraps, rolls etc that are made with flour that doesn't contain gluten.

If you discover gluten is a problem for you, it doesn't mean you have to break up with bread for good. You can cut down on how much you eat, and how often, or buy a gluten-free loaf instead.

Eggs

Chicken are not the only birds laying eggs apparently. You can replace chicken eggs with the eggs from quails, geese, ducks and ostriches. I've got absolutely no idea where you'd pick up a six-pack of ostrich eggs, so I'll leave it up to you to run about like a headless ehh….ostrich.

Small Adjustments, Not Big Life Changes

I'm not suggesting you completely banish any of the inflammatory foods I've listed. I certainly haven't. It can be a case of small adjustments, rather than big life changes, to help lower inflammation on a daily basis and keep you healthy and strong.

Here's how I've changed my own diet:

- I've completely eliminated peanuts and peanut butter. I simply eat almonds, pistachios, and almond butter instead.
- I try to cut out gluten as much as possible, avoiding pasta, bread, rolls etc. But I'll still have them a couple of times per week if I'm out for dinner, or the supermarket has run out of gluten-free bread.
- I stopped drinking cow's milk years ago, but the A2 milk is available at my local supermarket if I want it for tea/coffee.
- I've swapped normal cow's milk butter for French butter from grass-fed cows. It's a little bit more expensive, but tastes much better.

All of the above was easy to implement, and it's easy to maintain. I get fewer headaches than I used to, my stomach problems are well under control, and I feel much healthier now.

Lower inflammation = a stronger immune system, quicker recovery from workouts, fewer niggling health problems, and a healthier, better functioning you.

CHAPTER 10

Power Shakes That Pack A Nutritional Punch

So I was in bed after everything went to plan with the date. Girl came to my house, we got pissed drunk, had a laugh, ditched our clothes...and she was lying there next to me.

Life couldn't have been better, eh? Well actually, it could have.

Because the slight stomach cramps from the protein shake I'd drank a few hours earlier had gotten 1,000 times worse...and I was terrified I would actually shit the bed in my sleep.

That scene in Trainspotting flicked through my mind. The one where Spud comes downstairs with the bedsheets covered in the smelly stuff.

What was I going to do? Creep out of bed and just go to the toilet? No chance – the bathroom wall was right next to the bed and my rumbling belly felt like a volcano.

She would have heard the almighty explosion next door. My chances of another date would have gone right down the toilet pan.

"Guuuuuuurrrrgggglllllllllle........."– awww man, I couldn't believe the noises from my stomach hadn't woken her up.

But I decided I was going to have to wake her up now anyway.....because I only had minutes left.

*"You're going to have to go home now...."*I said as I shook her hurriedly.*"I can't get to sleep with someone else in the bed."*

*"But it's 6.30am,"*she said.

"I know but I start work in just a few hours and need to get at least some sleep."

*"Fine!"*she replied as she threw on her clothes and walked downstairs for what seemed like 17 years.

As soon as I shut the front door behind her, I turned into some sort of Olympic acrobat. I leapt over my sofa, flew upstairs, pulled down my boxer shorts and landed on the toilet pan...all in one flawless sequence.

I'd made it. But I came within seconds of destroying my boxer shorts, credibility...and toilet cistern.

The moral of the story: be careful about what kind of protein shakes you have - and don't drink two of them before going on a date.

This whole incident happened nearly five years ago after I bought a tub of protein powder mixed with creatine, and a few extras supposed to help the muscle building and recovery process.

This supplement was produced by a big-name brand but it was sickly sweet when I first tasted it, and when I looked on the back of the container there was a huge list of ingredients (many of which I'd never heard of before).

These were warning signs that I'd bought a product that should probably be poured straight into the bin, rather than down my throat. I didn't pay attention and, after drinking two shakes on that fateful day, I felt sick, nauseous, and...well, I won't repeat the toilet trouble story.

Ever since then I've only bought basic protein powder supplements that are natural, organic, easy to digest, and don't include any dodgy chemicals or additives I've never heard of.

More importantly, it inspired me to create my own type of protein shakes/healthy smoothies with a bunch of all-natural, healthy ingredients that I have handpicked.

I call them 'power shakes' because they pack a real punch – and contain more vitamins, minerals and other nutrients in one single shake than most people will consume over the course of an entire day.

They're also anti-inflammatory, of course, making it easier for your body to absorb all the nutrients.

I'm going to share with you the benefit of introducing these power shakes into your diet, the ideal time to drink them, and how they can help you maximize results from your workouts. I'll then list a couple of my favourite recipes, which are simple to make and taste outrageously good.

Supplying Your Body With The Tools It Needs

It is harder than ever to provide your body with the proper tools to do its job in keeping you healthy, strong and happy.

By 'tools' I'm talking vitamins, minerals, amino acids, essential fatty acids, phytonutrients etc. Going beyond protein, carbs and fats, and considering these all-important micronutrients at a smaller level that keep us alive and kicking.

For example, there are 13 essential vitamins and 16 essential minerals that are considered crucial to the healthy functioning of our bodies.

Government health agencies, such as the FDA in the US, tell us that the recommended daily allowance of vitamins and minerals. For example, vitamin A is 5,000 IU, while the minimum amount of calcium is 1,000mg.

Vitamin A is important for immune system function, your vision, red blood cell formation, and your skin and bones. Calcium plays several important roles including developing strong teeth and bones, supporting nervous system function, and muscle contraction.

The idea is that if your diet includes a wide variety of foods, including fresh fruit and vegetables, nuts, seeds, meats etc, then you'll be getting the vitamins and minerals your body needs.

That may have been true decades ago, but these days we are generally taking in fewer micronutrients than we used to. This is due to several reasons:

- **Intensive farming** – the demand on farmers to produce more and more for a growing world population, along with the use of pesticides and fertilizers, has resulted in depleted soils. This means fewer vitamins and minerals in today's fruit and vegetables.

- **Processed foods** – our supermarkets shelves are filled with foods that have additives, preservatives, and are processed to the point where they're stripped of their natural vitamins and minerals.

- **Overcooking** – heat in the cooking process also reduces the nutrient levels in your vegetables and fruit. Okay, none of us want to eat a raw cabbage, but overcooking can leave you with a less healthy plate of vegetables than you expected.

The simple point I'm making is that in our Western society hitting these recommended daily amounts isn't as easy as it looks. And many health experts believe that the recommended intake for some vitamins and minerals should actually be considerably higher.

Chronic deficiencies lead to niggling health problems, and will hamper your efforts to get in great shape because the body simply doesn't have the tools it needs to do many important jobs including converting food into energy, repairing cellular damage, and building muscle tissue.

Plenty Of Nutrients Packed Into One Shake

Given the importance of micronutrients for hitting your fitness goals, and your overall health, it makes sense to take additional steps to plug the gaps left by the 'Standard American Diet'.

Taking a quality multivitamin and mineral supplement daily is definitely a good move. It's also a brilliant idea to whizz yourself up a super nutritious power shake each day, which also has the additional calories, protein, carbs and fats needed to strengthen and develop your body.

I recommend making a power shake filled with fruit, protein powder, a little veg, nuts, and spices your first 'meal' of the day. Below I've listed four reasons why:

- **It's a nutritional powerhouse** – you'll struggle to find any main meal on the planet that includes such a wide variety of nutritious foods. The beauty of a shake is that you can simply throw them all together in the blender, whizz them up, and then you're good to go.
- **It's quick and easy** – it literally takes 2 mins to create one of these shakes. Much easier and convenient than cooking a breakfast or making a packed lunch for work.
- **You retain the goodness** – making a shake requires no boiling, baking or cooking of any sort. You can throw in fruit and veg straight from the freezer, which not only preserves the vitamins and minerals, but retains a fuller flavour.
- **Better nutrient absorption** – by using a host of whole, natural ingredients, and blending them up into a liquid meal, you make the job breaking down and absorbing the nutrients from your food much easier for your digestive system.

I make a power shake my first meal of the day most days of the week. Almost always Monday to Friday, and then mix things up a little at the weekend – just incase I turn into the most predictable, boring, shake-slurper in Scotland.

The reason for having making it meal number one is that it eases your body back into the digestion process after a long lay-off during sleep etc.

I don't know about you, but if I have a typical big breakfast filled with eggs, sausages, beans, bacon, toast etc, it makes me feel heavy and in need of another sleep.

An easily-digestible power shake not only gives you plenty of energy and nutrients for the day ahead, but it gives your stomach an easy warm-up ahead of heavier meals, such as a three-course dinner in the evening.

My Top 3 Power Shake Recipes

These simply involve a basic blender/food processor that you can buy for fairly cheap online. Add all ingredients, blend for 30 secs, and then pour into a 1 litre shaker cup.

Below I've listed my top three power shake recipes, along with a nutritional breakdown (although this will vary slightly based on which type of protein powder you use). I use Sun Warrior's Warrior Blend, chocolate flavour.

Choc N' Blueberry

- Handful of frozen blueberries
- ½ frozen banana

- 2 small pieces of frozen broccoli
- 1 scoop of chocolate protein powder
- 1/4 can / 100ml of coconut milk
- 3 tbsp of milled linseed
- Handful of almonds
- 1 tsp of cinnamon powder
- ¾ pint of water

Nutritional Breakdown

- Calories: 620
- Protein: 30g
- Carbohydrates: 29g
- Fat: 43g
- Fibre: 14g

- Vitamin C: 70% RDA
- Iron: 34%
- Calcium: 6% RDA
- Potassium: 25%
- Sodium: 30%

Mango & Pineapple

- Handful of frozen mango chunks
- Handful of frozen pineapple chunks

- A few leaves of spinach
- 1 scoop of chocolate protein powder
- 1/4 can / 100ml of coconut milk
- 3 tbsp of milled linseed
- Handful of almonds
- 1 tsp of ground ginger
- ¾ pint of water

Nutritional Breakdown (numbers may vary slightly)

- Calories: 658
- Protein: 31g
- Carbohydrates: 32g
- Fat: 42g
- Fibre 13g

- Vitamin A: 67% RDA
- Vitamin C: 74% RDA
- Iron: 38% RDA
- Calcium: 7% RDA
- Potassium: 8% RDA
- Sodium: 26% RDA

Strawberry & Banana

- Handful of frozen strawberries
- ½ frozen banana
- 2 small pieces of frozen broccoli
- 1 scoop of chocolate protein powder
- 1 tbsp of almond butter
- 3 tbsp of milled linseed
- 1 tsp of ground ginger
- ¾ pint of water

Nutritional Breakdown (numbers may vary slightly)

- Calories: 443
- Protein: 29g
- Carbohydrates: 32g
- Fat: 22g
- Fibre: 16g

- Vitamin A: 1% RDA
- Vitamin C: 104% RDA
- Iron: 34% RDA
- Calcium: 9% RDA
- Potassium: 42% RDA
- Sodium: 24% RDA

Simple to follow. Quick to make. Tasty as hell.

Oh, and incase you were wondering, I did get the second date with that girl. And after a few years of us being together, I confessed all about my toilet trouble that night.

CHAPTER 11

Anabolic Boosting Foods

As I sat in my cousin's bedroom with my eyes glued to the TV, my feelings of excitement were quickly replaced by a queasiness in my stomach.

It was the summer holidays and I was holed up in the loft of my aunt's house, which was converted to a bedroom for my big cousin Alistair.

As a 10-year-old boy, this was crazily exciting for me. I was sleeping in a room which was more like a 'den' in the roofspace of the house – and I didn't have to share a bedroom with my sister.

And just to complete my entire young existence, the Rocky movie was showing on TV. I was obsessed with the Sly Stallone boxing movies ever since I first watched Rocky IV.

There was something about him exercising in a ramshackle Russian barn in -150 degrees – with slightly cheesy 80s music playing in the background – that got me hooked.

Every time I watched the training scenes and heard the familiar trumpets in the 'Gonna Fly Now' song or the chords for 'Heart's On Fire', my heart would pump like mad, and it'd make me want work out, build muscle, become strong as fuck, and then feel as superhuman as my main man Sly.

I was working my way backwards through the Rocky series and had tuned into the original movie, from 1976, at my aunt's house.

Everything was going to plan.

A big fight lined up with the heavyweight champ of the world. Check.

Training scenes with Rocky running through the streets of Philadelphia as lots of random kids chase him. Check.

Compulsory motivational music to accompany said training montage. Check.

Then something happened that wasn't in the usual script. A scene I wasn't expecting...

It was 4.01am and Rocky reached up to switch off the rattling alarm clock above his bed. He spinned off the mattress and shivered in the cold winter morning.

Then he stepped forward, grabbed an egg from the fridge, and cracked it straight into a glass. Then another egg, then another, and then another one.

At this point I was a bit confused. I was thinking he should've had his training shoes on faster than a three-punch Apollo Creed combo. He should've been outside beginning his 50-mile morning run with the milkman, cockerels, and whoever else was awake at that time chasing him through the streets.

Instead he was messing about cracking eggs into a glass. I mean, what was the point in breaking them into a glass? Surely it should've been a frying pan instead? Surely he wasn't going to drink all that gooey, translucent, orange-spotted slime?

And he did.

And the yolk also did drip down his chin onto his light grey cotton jumper. My stomach was scrambled. My 10-year-old brain was fried.

What the hell was Rocky doing? I thought he just had to run for miles, do lots of sparring, and workout in the gym like a warrior to become a heroic heavyweight champ of the world.

I was ready to set my alarm early and do all of that hard, sweaty work to become just like Rocky.

I definitely wasn't ready to gag on a half-pint of slimey, raw eggs every morning.

I remember telling my mum about this horrifying scene in the movie, and was surprised when she informed me that my grandfather used to do the same thing.

"He'd mix up two or three raw eggs in a cup and then quickly swallow it," she explained. "He said it kept him strong and healthy."

Turns out Rocky, my grandad, and even spinach-munching Popeye were ahead of the game!

They were all eating these foods because of the anabolic (aka muscle building) effects they have on the body. There are a variety of foods you can include in your diet that'll support the production of the anabolic hormones.

The good news: you don't have to guzzle 35 raw eggs every week. It's also not necessary to have yolk dripping down your chin...or drying into a crispy, yellow stain on your clothes.

Let's now cover seven stupendous anabolic foods, not in any particular order, that can help build a stronger and healthier you.

Seven Stupendous Anabolic Foods

#1 You guessed it…eggs

Chicken eggs are considered a superfood by some health experts as they pack a huge amount of nutritional goodness within one shell.

Not only are eggs a great source of protein, they also contain healthy fatty acids, good cholesterol, along with numerous vitamins and minerals.

Don't be fooled by all the hype around egg whites, particularly in the health and fitness world where many people buy dried egg whites as a supplement. The fact is, most of the nutrition is in the yolk.

One large free-range egg contains approximately 6g of protein, 4.5g of fat (1.5g of saturated), and around 0.1g of carbohydrates. Chicken eggs supply all of the essential amino acids – the building blocks of protein needed for workout recovery and muscle development.

They also pack in various amounts of all these vitamins and minerals:

- **Vitamin A** (promotes skeletal growth, healthy skin, eyes and hair etc).

- **Vitamin B1** (helps convert sugar into energy, supports digestion, prevents fatigue etc).
- **Vitamin B2** (helps release energy to the cells, enables utilisation of fats, proteins and sugars).
- **Vitamin B5** (necessary for making blood cells, and also helps you convert food into energy).
- **Folic acid** (helps the body produce and maintain new cells).
- **Vitamin K** (plays a role in blood clotting, bone metabolism, and regulating calcium levels).
- **Choline** (support key neurotransmitters and helps process fat and cholesterol).
- **Calcium** (essential for muscle contraction, strong bones and teeth, blood clotting regulating heartbeat etc).
- **Iron** (vital to the proper function of haemoglobin, a protein needed to transport oxygen in the blood).
- **Phosphorus** (helps repair and build the body's cells and tissues).

Meanwhile, the cholesterol found in eggs has been shown to have a positive impact on levels of the anabolic hormone testosterone.

Research carried out in the 1980s involving more than 4,000 men demonstrated a "positive association" between higher levels of HDL cholesterol and total testosterone.

Opt for eggs from organic, pasture-raised hens as they are healthier and produce eggs that have a superior nutritional content than factory-raised hens.

#2 Asparagus

Those little green spears are one of the most nutritionally balanced plant foods. Asparagus provides a dose of potassium and folic acid, which aid in the production of chemicals that enhance sex drive. It also contains vitamin E, which stimulates the production of testosterone.

A half cup of cooked asparagus also contains around 60% of the RDI of vitamin K, 35% of the RDI of folate, almost 20% of the RDI of vitamin A, and roughly 12% of the RDI of vitamin C.

Asparagus also contains the mineral magnesium, which has many functions in the body, and studies have shown that magnesium intake affects the secretion of IGF-1 and increases testosterone bioactivity.

#3 Brazil nuts

Masses of guys have been going bonkers for Brazil nuts after Tim Ferriss released his book 'The 4 Hour Body'. He described a protocol, which included eating three Brazil nuts in the morning and another three before bed to raise testosterone levels.

Sounds a bit nuts, right? (See what I did there?) Maybe not, because Brazil nuts are the world's richest known source for the mineral selenium – and selenium has been linked to elevated testosterone levels.

A study was done at a fertility clinic in Nigeria in 2012 involving 50 fertile men and 25 infertile men. Researchers discovered big differences in the levels of selenium, zinc and testosterone between the two groups of men.

They concluded that there was a relationship between levels of selenium and zinc and the testosterone in the infertile men.

Stick to fewer than six Brazil nuts per day as excessive amounts of selenium can have unwanted side effects including nausea.

#4 Avocado

Okay, so they aren't quite as tasty as a ripe banana or juicy strawberries, but avocados are chock full of goodness that can also boost your anabolic hormones.

These bad boys are the only fruit that contains monounsaturated fat (a good kind) and 20 vitamins and minerals, including potassium, vitamin E, and the B vitamins.

Monounsaturated fats help maximise testosterone production, and support the production of other hormones in the body. They also improve cholesterol levels, reducing the risk of heart disease.

A medium-sized avocado also contains around 10g of fibre - around 40% of your RDI - helping to keep your digestion in good working order.

#5 Spinach

Popeye was clearly clued-up when it came to good nutrition, but I doubt if I'd munch on spinach straight out of a can like he did.

The leafy vegetable is also packed with lots of vitamins and minerals, but its muscle-building reputation made famous in Popeye is down to its plant-based steroids called 'phytoecdysteroids'.

These compounds keeps blood sugar levels stable and can increase muscle tissue growth by up to 20%, according to a study done in 2008.

#6 Quinoa

This South American seed is packed with ecdysterone, the same kind of natural steroid found in spinach.

A diet high in ecdysterone and protein can increase muscle mass by up to 7%, according to sports scientists.

It makes sense then to combine this super-seed with the likes of chicken or pork a few times per week.

#7 Cinnamon

You'll know from the previous chapter on inflammation-fighting foods that I'm a big fan of cinnamon. The fact that it tastes addictively good is a huge bonus.

I only recently discovered through fitness and hormone expert Mike Mahler that it has anabolic-boosting properties too.

After delving further into some research, I found that several studies have been done on rats (none yet on humans unfortunately) which suggest that cinnamon has a positive effect on the functioning of the body.

One particular study carried out in Egypt in 2010 caught my attention. Researchers looked closely at the effects of cinnamon and ginger on the fertility of diabetic rats. The results were that cinnamon at 500mg per kg of weight raised testosterone levels - and decreased blood sugar levels – providing an all-round health improvement.

CHAPTER 12

Intermittent Fasting For Easy Fat Loss

"Help out a brother!"

The message flashed up on my mobile phone like a desperate SOS plea. It was from my mate Chris, who I hadn't heard from in a while. What was up? Had something happened? Was he about to ask me for some serious life advice?

"I'm going on holiday to Turkey soon and really need to lose some weight soon," he wrote.

I was a bit surprised by this because I knew Chris was generally pretty fit, and lifted weights at the gym several times per week.

He still did. No problems on that front. The issues were in the diet department.

Chris had started dating a girl and the two of them were living it up in an extended honeymoon phase. Takeaway meals, too much wine, bags of sweet treats while going nuts for Netflix. You know the drill.

Chris had piled on around 25lbs and was the heaviest he'd ever been. The pair were due to fly out for a beach holiday in Turkey – and he was feeling like a giant Christmas Turkey.

"Okay no probs," I replied. "But how soon are you going on holiday?"

Chris wrote: "Ehhh...in under two weeks. Should I go to the gym every day until then? What should I cut out my diet? Can you give me one of your programmes?"

One of my training programmes lasted 10 weeks. Chris was after results closer to 10 days. Didn't exactly give me much to work with.

I'd been in the gym with Chris before that and he knew what he was doing. Apart from maybe a few tweaks to his weights sessions, his training routine was on point.

Chris's weight gain was all down to his poor diet, not inactivity. He wanted to <u>burn fat fast</u> – and just like in my book with the same title – my #1 piece of advice was to implement intermittent fasting.

For weight loss you don't have to...

Cut out carbs like crazy until you feel fatigued and fed-up.

Go on a juicing diet and guzzle disgusting tasting veggie smoothies day after day.

Ban all your favourite foods and become the most miserable person you know.

No, it's more straightforward than you think. Rather than putting all the focus on what you eat when trying to burn fat or hit a weight target, a better move is to also look closely at WHEN you eat.

That's at the core of intermittent fasting – and it can bring outstanding results. (As Chris discovered). Insert winking smiley face right here.

Intermittent fasting is without doubt my number one tactic for burning fat. I've seen it with work wonders with men and women of all ages, weights, and fitness levels.

I'm not talking about some sort of fad diet, or short-term fix. Intermittent fasting is a simple *lifestyle change* that is natural, easy to implement, and can have dramatic positive effects on your health.

Intermittent fasting enables your body to turn on the automatic fat burning switch, and it brings a whole host of other health benefits.

Best of all: it's really easy to introduce and maintain. I don't know you, but if you've struggled with excess flab, losing weight, or have been on yo-yo diets, then intermittent fasting might well be the answer to your prayers.

How Intermittent Fasting Works

Intermittent fasting – as you've probably already guessed from name – involves an extended break from food. It doesn't mean you'll be starving, but it also doesn't mean continuing with the breakfast, lunch, dinner...and snacks in between...standard way of eating.

By adjusting your eating habits, and having an extended break without food each day, you can give your body a signal to burn fat automatically. No exercise involved, no low-fat foods involved, no willpower struggle involved.

Here's how it works: your body's main source of energy is the glucose it derives from carbohydrates. Excess glucose is converted into glycogen and stored in the liver and muscle cells for a ready-made supply of energy later.

Think of it like a glycogen bank where your body takes deposits for energy throughout your day. But when that bank of glycogen runs out your body needs to look elsewhere for fuel.

Where's the first port of call? Your fat stores! In a process called lipolysis, the body breaks down the fat stored in your white adipose tissue into free fatty acids in the blood stream.

These released fatty acids are then used as your primary fuel source. How long does it take for your glycogen bank to run out?

Glad you asked. It generally takes 12-14 hours for you to reach this fasted state and for the amount of fatty acids in the bloodstream to increase. Between 18 and 24 hours the number of fatty acids increases even further.

Regularly going without food for 24 hours is obviously not going to end well. And you're probably thinking, 'how the hell am I going to last even 14 hours without food?'

It's much easier than you'd expect.

A New Way Of Eating That's Easy To Maintain

Intermittent fasting can be easily implemented and successfully maintained by putting these two words into practice: SKIP BREAKFAST.

Forget all the outdated crap you've heard about breakfast being 'the most important meal of the day'. That might be true for five-year-old children who demand a bowl of Coco Pops before even opening a book at school.

I'm guessing you're a fully-fledged, fully-grown adult that can easily avoid a meltdown without foods for a few more hours. We're not talking Jesus-style, 30 days and 30 nights in the desert without a single crumb of bread.

No, we're talking resisting a bacon roll and coffee in the morning, and hanging on in there until 1pm, or even 12noon, before you have your first feed of the day.

By doing this, you'll almost certainly switch from carbohydrates to bodyfat as your primary source of energy...and you'll be burning excess fat on automatic.

This is not dieting. Diets never last in the long run, and generally require a big dose of willpower to maintain.

Instead, intermittent fasting is a new way of eating. It simply involves skipping breakfast each day to give your body the chance to use up its fat stores, and generate several other health benefits (which we'll cover shortly).

But first, let's look at the ideal time period for intermittent fasting. I always recommend aiming for a period of 14-16 hours without food/drink, meaning that you eat within an 8-10 hour window each day.

This is the exact approach I take. It's flexible and means I'm not clock watching or eating to a strict schedule. Most days I'll finish eating between 7pm and 8pm, and I'll not usually eat again until around 11am or 12noon the following day.

This is a 16-hour break without food, and the beauty of it is that I've been sleeping through most of that period. Therefore, it's not a difficult task or some sort of mental battle each day to keep up. It simply involves waiting another four hours or so before I have my first meal of the day.

What if you get home from work late and don't finish your dinner till 9pm, or even 10pm? Easy, just hold off another hour or two the next day, and don't have your lunch until around 1pm or 2pm.

As long as you maintain a 14-16 hour gap between your last meal at night and first meal the following day, you're going to end up in the fat burning zone.

Important tip: follow intermittent fasting just 4-5 days per week, and eat normally on the other days. By switching things up, the body doesn't adapt and intermittent fasting maintains its effectiveness. Studies have shown that intermittent fasting in cycles produces better results in the long term.

Personally, I do intermittent fasting Monday-Friday, and have breakfast - as well as generally relaxing my diet - at the weekend. It keeps me lean effortlessly, while preserving muscle. I've also seen it produce great results with past fitness clients, family and friends.

Being a fitness author, I often get asked the best way to lose the love handles – and unwanted fat elsewhere on the body. My first response is usually: "Have you heard of intermittent fasting?"

I've lost count of the times people have messaged me saying things like, "it's only been a week and I've lost 4lbs already," or "I've lost another 2lbs and I can't believe how easy this is."

Most people who follow intermittent fasting tell me that they get used to this new way of eating within a week. Their stomach grumbles for the first two or three days, and then their body naturally adjusts; only getting hungry around the 14-16 hour mark.

Remember, this is the way our ancestors ate. Going back to the hunter-gatherer days, humans would typically be out for long chunks of the day hunting and foraging. Feasting wouldn't occur until the evening, meaning a long, extended break without food.

These days you only have to walk a few hundred yards in your local town to hunt down a double cheeseburger with fries, or a fried chicken covered in breadcrumbs. And forget waiting till night-time when you can get stuck into a KFC chicken bucket for breakfast.

Live Forever (Or Maybe Just A Bit Longer) With Intermittent Fasting

Rapid fat burning is only one of many reasons to introduce intermittent fasting into your life. Another is that it helps slow down the aging process because it stimulates the body to maintain and repair tissues more efficiently.

It's also believed that intermittent fasting causes a mild form of stress, which prompts the body to build up cellular defences against molecular damage.

In 1945, scientists at the University of Chicago reported that alternate-day feeding extended the life-span of rats. They added that intermittent fasting "seems to delay the development of the disorders that lead to death."

Below I'll briefly touch upon some other key benefits of intermittent fasting, but this is certainly not the complete list.

Protects against brain disorders

Mark Mattson, head of the US National Institute On Aging's neuroscience lab, has led several studies with rodents looking closely at the effects of periodic fasting on health.

His team discovered that intermittent fasting protects against stroke damage, suppresses motor issues in a mouse model of Parkinson's Disease, and slows down the cognitive decline of mice genetically engineered to have Alzheimer's symptoms.

Helps prevent killer diseases

Intermittent fasting can help ward off major diseases and control chronic conditions. Researchers underlined this huge potential in a scientific paper published in 2014.

They wrote: "In rodents intermittent or periodic fasting protects against diabetes, cancers, heart disease, and neuro-degeneration, while in humans it helps reduce obesity, hypertension, asthma, and rheumatoid arthritis.

"Thus, fasting has the potential to delay aging and help prevent and treat diseases, while minimizing the side effects caused by chronic dietary interventions."

Increases growth hormone levels

We already know that fat-busting, muscle developing role that growth hormone plays in the body. Some studies have shown that in men, levels of growth hormone may rise by up to five-fold.

A 1992 study involved nine men fasting over a two day period and their levels of growth hormone (GH) being recorded regularly.

They reported: "Two days of fasting included a five-fold increase in the 24 hour endogenous GH production rate."

Keeps your heart healthy

We already touched upon how intermittent fasting has been shown to reduce heart disease risk factors. But it has also shown to positive influence another heart health factor – cholesterol.

In one 2012 study, 102 people in the Far East who were fasting during Ramadan were studied one day after Ramadan ended, and again a month later.

The researchers discovered that levels of good cholesterol increased, while cholesterol had declined.

They wrote: "We observed significant improvements in HDL-C and LDL-C levels even after four weeks post Ramadan."

Reduces inflammation

As you know, bringing down inflammation levels in your body and brain is crucial for good health.

A study published in 2015 looked closely at the associations of eating frequency and timing with metabolic and inflammatory markers. This particular study involved women at risk of breast cancer who were taking part in a national health survey in the US.

The study concluded: "Eating more frequently, reducing evening energy intake, and fasting for longer nightly intervals may lower systemic inflammation and subsequently reduce breast cancer risk."

Improved sports performance

Intermittent fasting can lead to you performing better in your gym workouts, and in other sports. This is directly linked to the increase in growth hormone.

Elevated levels of growth hormone will not only strip away unwanted fat from your frame, but it'll trigger muscle growth and help you become stronger and fitter.

Detoxification

Our foods, environment, and sometimes even our drinking water can contain harmful chemicals, additives and pesticides that can lead to a build-up of toxins in your system.

I don't mean to sound like some sort of Greenpeace hippy and suggest you eat nothing but organic vegetables and sparkling mineral water straight off the nearest mountain waterfall.

But it's a fact that if you become overloaded with too many toxins your immune system will suffer, and you'll become rundown and sick.

Intermittent fasting gives your body a helping hand because the break from all sorts of food also gives your digestive system a break. This allows your body to focus fully on clearing out unwanted toxins.

There you go, plenty of reasons to ditch breakfast and feel the benefits of intermittent fasting. Remember, 14-16 hours is an ideal fasting period that can be maintained effectively daily. Continuously fasting for longer periods than this may have actually slow down your metabolism.

As for my mate Chris, he ditched breakfast each day in the run up to his holiday. I also advised him to cut back on chocolate and sugary treats.

The result? He lost 10lbs in 10 days.

His weight at the end of the week-long holiday in the sunshine with booze, ice cream, and eating out every night? That figure on the scales still hasn't been disclosed...

CHAPTER 13

The Fat Loss Con That's Keeping You Fat – And Sick

Remember when every second advertisement on the TV used to be about "low fat" this and "low fat" that.

As if that was the answer to everyone's slimming dreams. They did it with yoghurts, ice cream, microwave meals, and all sorts of foods to make you think they were healthier – and make you buy.

What they didn't tell you was that while they were stripping away the fat from these foods, they were adding in sugar, salt and other unnecessary extras to replace the natural flavour that had been lost.

What they didn't tell you was that not all fat is bad, and in fact the much-demonised saturated fat is actually very important for immune health, brain health, stronger bones, and proper nerve-signalling in the body.

I cover the topic of fats in more detail in my book *Strength Training Nutrition 101*, so there's no point in me going on a long-winded fat rant right now.

The point I'm making is that we seem to be past the whole "low fat" craze now. You don't see half as many of those adverts on the TV and I'm assuming it's because people are simply more clued-up that most of these "low fat" processed foods are garbage.

The idea that these nutritionally-spent foods was the healthiest way to lose weight was a huge marketing con. It's a con that's largely gone away, at least where I live in the UK.

But there's another con that's still going strong. One that I doubt will ever go away in my lifetime. I'm talking about the whole "diet", "zero calories", and "no sugar" craze with drinks and food.

I'm not singling out any particular brand. You see it everywhere with fizzy juice, teas and coffees, shakes, and supposedly healthy foods.

We know sugar is bad for us and so the food and drinks manufacturers strip that out. Thumbs up. But then, just like with the processing of low fat foods, they throw in something that's worse!

Two words: artificial sweeteners.

There's a massive misconception across America, UK, Europe and beyond that these types of sweeteners are good for us. That they'll help us lose weight. That they're healthy and a much better option to sugar.

They're absolutely not.

When I worked in an office years ago I can remember making tea and coffee in the morning, and my workmates would be passing me their mugs – along with their little sweetener dispensers.

After pouring the hot water and adding the milk to 6 or 7 mugs, I'd then hover over the top of most of them and click once or twice until these tiny white sweeteners hit the water.

To me, they looked like little drug tablets of some kind, which initially put me off. But I also couldn't get my head around how something so tiny could have such a strong effect on the flavour of the tea/coffee. It would turn it super sweet, but in a weird-tasting way.

Back then, there was less research into the effects of artificial sweeteners on the body and I had no clue about where they came from or how they were made. I just didn't like the taste and my version of going healthier with tea was to take one sugar, instead of two.

Glad I did. I also never drank fizzy juice – which is loaded with sweeteners - but that doesn't mean that I escaped them completely. Sweeteners were also in the supposedly-healthier protein powder I'd been using for years, and they were also in some foods that I ate regularly.

Let's now look at the production of sweeteners, the effects they have on the body, why you should consider reducing them in your diet, and healthy alternatives you can easily introduce instead.

Six Artificial Sweeteners – And 600 Times Sweeter Than Sugar

The Food and Drug Administration (FDA) in America has approved six 'high-intensity' artificial sweeteners: saccharin, sucralose, acesulfame, aspartame, advantame and neotame.

Some health experts believed that by using artificial sweeteners in foods and drinks people could experience the same taste as sugar - but without the added calories. Fewer calories would mean fewer weight problems, and then we'd all live happily ever after in a world of artificial sweetness.

It hasn't quite worked out that way. While the calories may be missing, some of these artificially-made sweeteners are hundreds of times sweeter than table sugar.

That fact alone should have been ringing alarm bells after these sugar substitutes started making an appearance on supermarket shelves in the 1980s.

In an eye-opening CBS News report in 2004, a senior clinical nutritionist from the New York University Medical Centre, revealed the strength of these chemical sweeteners in some of America's top brands.

One, which contained aspartame, was 160 to 200 times sweeter than sugar. Another, with saccharin, was 300 to 500 times sweeter than sugar. And the third leading brand, which contained sucralose, was 600 times sweeter.

While the FDA and American Dietetic Association (ADA) acknowledge these are chemicals, they have passed them fit for human consumption and believe they can form part of healthy diet.

However, critics of the use of artificial sweeteners argue that the strength of these products interfere with the way we taste food, and it may make less intensely sweet foods, such as healthy fruit, unappealing.

In other words, the use of artificial sweeteners to avoid sugary, unhealthy junk food may inadvertently lead to you avoiding healthy, nutritious foods.

Science Catching Up With Artificial Sweeteners

Those super sugar substitutes that are supposed to help with weight loss may well do the opposite, research shows. One extended piece of researched, called the San Antonio Heart Study, analysed the relationship between drinking artificially-sweetened beverages and long term weight gain.

Researchers looked the weight of more than 5,000 men and women living in San Antonio, Texas, many of whom drank sweetened drinks regularly. Seven to eight years later, almost 4,000 people still alive and still living in the area, were re-examined.

It was discovered that those who drank 21 or more artificially-sweetened drinks per week almost doubled their overweight/obesity markers compared with those who drank none.

The researchers concluded: "These findings raise the question whether AS (artificial sweeteners) use might be fuelling – rather than fighting – our escalating obesity epidemic."

How Artificial Sweeteners Negatively Impact Your Health

Not only are these sugar alternatives keeping us fat, they're also making us sick. New research has shown that they can wreak havoc with your digestive system, and heighten your risk of developing some serious health conditions.

Artificial sweeteners can potentially wipe out the 'good' gut bacteria in your digestive tract, according to recent studies. This can negatively impact your overall health.

Good bacteria plays a critical role in the final absorption of nutrients, it can prevent allergies, prevent yeast and pathogens from spreading in the gut, and fend off inflammatory bowel disease.

Your gut is made up of around 100 trillion of these microscopic bacteria - good guys and bad guys. The problems occur when the bad guys start taking over and things get out of balance. Too much bad bacteria in the gut can lead to a multitude of health problems, and will affect your body's absorption from foods.

Your gut flora can boost the immune system and protects against invaders in various ways. A healthy balance of gut bacteria strengthens the defences of the gut wall and competes with pathogens for space and food. It also helps regulate the inflammatory immune response in the body.

Bottom line: you want to preserve the good bacteria in your gut, and help it flourish with probiotic rich foods.

Artificial sweeteners have the opposite effect, new research suggests. A study first published in the medical journal Molecules in 2018 involved university experts testing the toxicity of the six sweeteners approved by the FDA.

Lab tests showed that when exposed to just 1 milligram per millilitre of the artificial sweeteners, the bacteria found in the digestive system became toxic.

And a study where mice were fed the sweetener neotame for four weeks resulted in good bacteria being killed off in their guts, and microbiome being "significantly" altered.

Just like excessive consumption of the sugar they're supposed to replace, artificial sweeteners also increase your risk of developing type II diabetes.

A large scale study was carried out in France involving more than 66,000 women and it looked at their consumption of fruit juice, sugar drinks, and artificially-sweetened drinks.

While the fruit juice was associated with a decreased risk of type II diabetes, the artificially-sweetened drinks almost doubled the risk of developing the disease.

The researchers concluded: "A high consumption of artificially-sweetened beverages (603ml or more per week) was associated with significant greater risk of diabetes compared with that for non-consumers."

Metabolic syndrome is a group of connected conditions including high blood pressure, high blood sugar levels, worrying cholesterol levels, and excess bodyfat around the midsection. And guess what?

It has been linked numerous times to the over-consumption of fizzy drinks that are loaded with artificial sweeteners.

A study published in the journal Diabetic Care in 2009 showed a direct link between diet soda consumption and metabolic syndrome and diabetes.

The experts concluded: "At least daily consumption of diet soda was associated with a 36% greater relative risk of incident metabolic syndrome and a 67% greater relative risk of incident type 2 diabetes compared with non-consumption."

So What's The Healthy Alternative?

Stevia is a natural sweetener made from the stevia plant and has long been used in Asia in South America. It is now growing in popularity elsewhere across the world because it's low in calories and has health benefits including helping your body to absorb glucose.

While stevia is nearly 200 times sweeter than sugar, it doesn't raise your blood sugar levels and doesn't leave a nasty aftertaste.

The best version is the sweet leaf natural stevia which you can find on Amazon.

There are now several stevia-based sweeteners on the market too, which use purified extracts from the leaves of the stevia plant called 'steviol glycosides'.

These are the second-best option because they go through extra processing and are not all natural, however they're still a better alternative to the common artificial sweeteners found in the supermarkets.

My advice is cut out all fizzy drinks completely – whether they say "sugar free", "zero", or "diet" – and stop putting sweeteners in your tea and coffee.

Using just a little sugar instead or, even better, switching to green/herbal teas would be a sweeter move for your health and fitness.

CHAPTER 14

Delay Your Post-Workout Meal

It was just me and the man mountain in the gym changing room, and I began to feel a bit uneasy about what he was up to.

He'd finished his weights workout at around the same time as me, marched straight to his locker, and fished out his gym bag.

Reaching deep into the sports rucksack, he began rooting around inside. I wasn't sure exactly what he was after, but he clearly wanted to find it fast. He rustled his hand around, and again, and then muttered something to himself in a pissed-off tone.

"Did you forget your protein shake mate?" I said, trying to kickstart a casual conversation and ease the big dude's frustration.

"Ehhh...no, no. It's not that."

He swivelled his arm around a bit deeper in the bag and then I heard an unexpected, but familiar sound. It was like the rustle of a packet of crisps.

For about 1.2 seconds of my life in that gym changing room I was completely confused. Was this big muscleman with biceps bigger than my head ready to much on an unhealthy packet of cheese and onion crisps after his workout?

Surely, he was defeating the purpose of all his hard work in the gym? But before I got the chance to answer the question in my own head, he whipped his arm out of the rucksack and revealed a packet of...

Jelly beans.

This happened about five or six years ago, and it led me to discover why some super serious weightlifters/bodybuilders will eat a few sweets like jelly beans or gummy bears immediately after their workout.

The idea is all about ingesting a fast-acting sugar that'll spike your insulin levels effectively and supposedly help transport nutrients to your muscles quickly, i.e. if those jelly beans are followed immediately by a protein shake.

I've heard some other PTs tout this method to their clients, and I've seen some guys promote it on online fitness forums. At this same time, I've seen it ridiculed by many other experienced gym-goers with an in-depth knowledge of nutrition and physiology.

I'm with the latter crowd. In fact, I preach the opposite approach when it comes to post-workout nutrition.

No jelly beans. No gummy bears. No racing against the clock to guzzle every last drop of a protein shake down your neck immediately after the gym.

Instead, you should wait 60-90 mins before you have that post-workout meal. Hold off that little bit longer - and you can reap big fat burning and muscle building benefits.

Why You Should Hold Off On Your Post-Workout Meal

It all comes down to your glycogen levels and hormones once again. Breaking it all down to a basic level, there are two main reasons for waiting 60-90 mins before having your post-workout meal or shake.

#1 It keeps you in an anabolic state for longer

There's a window following your workout where glycogen levels are re-filled at a faster rate. This is to overcompensate for all the energy expended during your training session.

This is why you'll see tennis stars munch on bananas, or have sports drinks, in between sets. They're refilling their glycogen with simple sugar foods that can be quickly converted into glucose for energy. Their bodies top up their glycogen bank too, and they get sufficient fuel to get through long matches.

It's the way to go in a long endurance test like tennis, or possibly if you intend on hitting the gym hard day after day.

If you've read any of my previous books, you'll know that I recommend not doing this. I've long argued that one day on, one day off is the best approach when it comes to lifting weights for proper recovery, avoiding injury and overall health.

But, another downside to ingesting a sugary protein shake, or healthy meal, soon after your workouts is that it slows down the production of anabolic hormones. When insulin levels rise as a natural result of consuming your post-workout meal, your anabolic hormone levels decrease.

World renowned sports nutrition expert and author Mark Sisson, of marksdailyapple.com, has been helping design supplements for leading brands for over 30 years.

Mark is a big-name proponent of the ketogenic diet – and of fasting post-workout. In an interview on the awesome Joe Rogan podcast in 2016, Mark discussed the benefits of holding off on eating for 60-90 minutes after training. He gives an example of doing this after a tough legs weights session.

He said: "When you fast post-workout you don't replenish the glycogen, but you preserve the pulse of growth hormone and testosterone that happens as a result of leg day...which you would otherwise blunt by taking in a sugary drink.

"Insulin has an effect on growth hormone and testosterone. It actually lowers it.

"If you are eating a post-workout meal that's high in carbs because you want to refill the glycogen stores – so you can do it again tomorrow – then the post-workout meal will cause a rise in insulin, which will blunt the growth hormone and testosterone pulse that you got from that workout.

"But you'll have glycogen stores slightly more ready for another workout tomorrow. What are you trying to accomplish here?

"I'd rather just do the workout really hard, get all of the growth benefits I'm looking for, and not have to do it again tomorrow!"

#2 You'll burn even more fat

When you bust your ass in the gym and come out of there sweating like a maniac, the fat burning job is done. Right?

Wrong. It's basically only half done as exercise simply begins the fat breakdown process. Lots of free fatty acids that have been released from your white adipose tissue are still floating around in your bloodstream, and there are two ways they could go.

One – they could be mobilised to the liver and muscle to be metabolised. Two – they could be re-esterified into triglycerides and re-deposited back into your fat tissue.

The latter occurs when you consume your post-workout shake/meal too soon after training. Essentially, you're not making the most of your hard-earned gym efforts.

American fitness guru Dr Chad Waterbury and sports nutrition expert Ori Hofmekler cover this in more detail in this fascinating interview titled 'The Truth About Post Workout Nutrition'.

You can check it out by visiting: http://chadwaterbury.com/the-truth-about-post-workout-nutrition/

Personally, my approach is:

- Work out on an empty stomach in the morning.
- Wait 60-90 mins after my workout and drink one of the power shakes I described earlier. (Approx 10am-11am).
- Have a healthy lunch around 1pm-2pm, and dinner around 7pm.
- Take the next day off the gym, and then repeat the above the following day.

No point in getting overwhelmed with all this pre-workout and post-workout nutrition advice.

No point in complicating the uncomplicated.

And no need to be munching on jelly beans in any gym changing room.

RECOVERY & HEALTH OPTIMISATION

CHAPTER 15

Embrace The Cold

In the first part of this book there was a whole lot of heat...

From the in-depth look at inflammation in the body. From the inflammatory response caused by exercise and injury. And from the fires that can burn inside as a result of certain problem foods.

When those fires burn too high for too long we've got a problem. Not only can chronic inflammation hamper your fitness performance, it runs down your immune system and it can lead to disease.

In this section on recovery and health optimisation we're going to call in the firefighters. Yes, while those fires may burn in your body as a result of injury, stress, poor diet, infection etc, you can also take steps to douse the flames and keep them at low levels every single day.

This chapter and the next will explore two of the most effective methods that are known to man for bringing down inflammation naturally. I should know…they helped reverse my inflammatory bowel disease.

The cause and the cure of this disease were completely unexpected. I'll briefly explain what happened.

On December 8th, 2017, we got the shock news that my dad had died. He was aged 54 years old and was alone in his home when he passed away.

My mum crumbled and my priority was to help her through it all. I spoke with the police, the funeral directors, and took charge of organising every part of the funeral, from collecting the death certificate and organising the time of the service to copying CDs of the music to be played at the funeral.

I've always been a very organised person and so I treated this horrible time in our lives like any other important event that required a to-do list. I ticked off one task then another, without really letting my dad's death properly sink in.

The automatic pilot switch was turned on and I became busy as a distraction to what was really going on. I know many people reading this will be able to relate.

I cried a little at the funeral, but not much before or after it. I was fine, I was staying strong for my mum. I could handle everything. I had my shit together.

Or so I thought.

About a week after the funeral I'd hit the floor. The sadness and grief I'd tried to bury overflooded. Then my physical health took a nosedive. I was losing weight, looking pale, and my digestive system went into meltdown.

I was sprinting to the toilet within 15 minutes of finishing a meal. Up during the night with diarrhoea two or three times a night. But the worst part was the bleeding.

I'd had stomach problems on and off for several years, but I always managed to keep it under control with a healthy diet. I'd never experienced anything like this and the regular bleeding was getting me worried.

I went into hospital for another colonoscopy procedure, which I was dreading. The last time they prodded around up there with the little camera on a stick it was agony – and it lasted for what seemed like an hour.

This time the ordeal was over in just a minute, as the nurse told me: "You have ulcerative colitis, Marc. Your lower colon is pretty badly inflamed and ulcerated. But don't worry, we'll prescribe steroids and other medication."

I walked home slowly with the letter I was to take to the pharmacist, and read the words: "Moderate to severe ulcerative colitis."

It sounded pretty serious, but I was just pleased that they'd figured out what was wrong with me. I also couldn't wait to get my hands on the medication that I hoped would stop the bleeding and get my health back on track.

I understood *what* had happened. My lower colon had become badly inflamed, and remained that way for so long that disease took hold. But I couldn't get my head around *why* it had happened.

I followed a healthy diet and, while I did eat some inflammatory foods, I wasn't overdoing it. I'd exercised regularly for over 20 years, I didn't smoke, and I barely drank alcohol. As a health and fitness trainer, I was always preaching about healthy living and taking care of your body...and yet I was ill with a serious disease.

None of it made sense. Well, until I started doing more research into colitis and its causes. I soon discovered that emotional trauma, such as the death of a relative, can trigger the onset of colitis.

The emotional stress, particularly when much of it is suppressed, can lead to high levels of inflammation in the body. This is exactly what happened with me and it was my lower colon that suffered.

I was given steroids (not the same anabolic ones dodgy bodybuilders use) for a month to bring down the inflammation, as well as another anti-inflammatory drug called mesalazine, which I was told I'd likely have to take indefinitely.

The drugs worked a treat and most of my symptoms had died down after just a couple of weeks. While both those drugs were very important in helping me regain my health, I didn't feel comfortable with the idea of taking an anti-inflammatory drug every day for the long term.

By pure chance, I found out that I didn't have to.

Six months later, I went on holiday to Waterloo in Canada to visit my aunt and cousins. Everything went to plan...good weather for two weeks, good food, and great company.

But there was one problem: I didn't have my medication with me. I tried to pick up my mesalazine supply on the way to the airport, but the pharmacist messed up my prescription and it wasn't going to be ready on time. I had to leave empty-handed – or I would've missed my flight.

I treated the holiday exactly like you should treat a holiday...eating and drinking lots of what you don't normally eat and drink. I was munching on hot dogs, peanut butter and chocolate chip cookies, sugary drinks, and BBQ food basically every night.

I would NEVER do this back home, but randomly went on a junk food frenzy simply because I was on a two week break with relatives I hadn't seen for years.

It got to day 11 of the holiday before it all caught up with me. I woke up that morning with a pounding headache, feeling sick, and there was a little blood again when I went to the toilet.

I instantly knew what it meant. No medication + non-stop junk food + my delicate digestive system = high inflammation again.

This time I couldn't just pick up my medication to get things under control again, and the hospital and pharmacist were over 3,000 miles away. I wouldn't be home for another three days so I had to find a plan B for feeling better.

The first and most obvious thing to do was stop eating all the junk food. My body simply wasn't used to it in small amounts, never mind 11 days of gorging like a kid in a chocolate factory.

Then, after flicking through some videos on YouTube, I came across Wim Hof again. I'd first stumbled across this crazy Dutchman earlier in the year and was intrigued by his extraordinary approach for maintaining health, strength and wellness.

I'm going to dive much deeper into the Wim Hof Method in the next chapter, but for now I'll focus on one important element of his approach for health and wellness...

Cold therapy. In simpler terms: cold showers every day.

Cold Showers Will Make You Healthier And Stronger

It doesn't sound like much fun, and it isn't. However, repeatedly exposing your body to the cold naturally helps cool the heat within your tissues and organs.

Taking cold showers has been scientifically proven to bring down inflammation within the body, helping you to recover from workouts and injuries, improve your health, and even have a positive impact on your mental state.

There are many other benefits to taking cold showers regularly, which include enhancing your immune system, improving blood circulation, and stimulating the production of more anabolic hormones.

Author and speaker Paul Chek, who is a world-renowned expert in strength and conditioning and holistic wellness, is a big fan of cold showers for health and healing.

In an online with Underground Wellness, he said: "We have a world full of people that are inflamed to the hilt on the inside and outside. They run around doctors and therapists...and all you've got to do is jump in a cold shower.

"It conditions your autonomic nervous system, it exercises the arterial vascular tree, it aids in your ability to regulate your inner temperature relative to the environment, it stimulates the immune system, it has anabolic effects and improves your sex life...it's free!

"And what do you get? 'Oh I could never take a cold shower...'

"You get people who would rather have their organs cut out than take a cold shower. Well, as a therapist, that just tells me that their autonomic nervous system is extremely weak."

Thousands of people across the world practicing the Wim Hof Method incorporate cold showers into their daily routine. They report back that they experience reduce levels of stress, high alertness and concentration, a stronger immune system, more willpower, and even weight loss.

One huge benefit that really caught my attention is that cold showers can even increase your happiness! A 2007 published by a molecular biologist named Nikolai Shevcuk found evidence that cold showers can help treat depression. This is down to the cold water sparking a rush of mood-boosting neurotransmitters in the brain.

In the study, Shevcuk reported: "Exposure to cold is known to activate the sympathetic nervous system and increase the blood level of beta-endorphin and noradrenaline, and to increase synaptic release of noradrenaline in the brain as well.

"Additionally, due to the high density of cold receptors in the skin, a cold shower is expected to send an overwhelming amount of electrical impulses from peripheral nerve endings to the brain, which could result in an anti-depressive effect.

"Practical testing by a statistically insignificant number of people, who did not have sufficient symptoms to be diagnosed with depression, showed that the cold hydrotherapy can relieve depressive symptoms rather effectively."

7 Other Brilliant Benefits Of Cold Showers

#1 Building mental strength

Cold showers are not fun. Especially on a winter morning when the water pipes are almost frozen - and you're still half-sleeping.

I'll be honest, my mind goes into overdrive nearly every time I'm getting ready for a shower, coming up with endless excuses to avoid the cold setting.

"It's the weekend, give yourself a wee break…." or "have a nice warm shower now, and you can maybe have a cold shower after the gym later."

By overcoming your own excuses and doing what's uncomfortable you strengthen your willpower, resilience, and set the tone for a productive day.

#2 You can handle stress better

No matter how well organised and focused we are, we all get hit with unimaginable, unexpected crap some days. These stressful incidents can easily throw us off track – and be the difference between a great day and a grim day.

But with cold showers you come prepared. You've already faced something you didn't want to face, and the slight shock to the system helps harden you to what life can throw at you next.

A 1999 study with winter swimmers shows that the cold acts as a smaller form of oxidative stress on your nervous system, which the body adapts to over time. Thus cold showers will help you handle stress in a cooler, calmer way.

#3 Healthier skin and hair

I thought it was an old wives' tale that rinsing hair with cold water made it shinier. Turns out there's real evidence that it makes your hair and skin healthier.

Cold water helps prevent your hair and skin from losing too many natural oils. It initially helps constrict blood vessels in your skin to temporarily tighten pores and reduce puffiness and redness.

Cold showers can also make hair shinier and stronger by flattening hair follicles, and increasing their ability to grip the scalp.

#4 Stimulates weight loss

There are two types of fat in the body: white and brown. White fat is the bad stuff that gathers where we don't want it, and leaves us out of shape.

Brown fat, however, is good for us. It generates heat in the body and helps keep us warm. Taking cold showers activates brown fat, which leads to an increase in energy and calories being burned.

#5 Drains your lymphatic system

The lymphatic system is like your body's sewer network. It carries waste out of the cells, however if your lymphatic system gets blocked then it's likely you'll get sick with colds, infections etc.

By blasting your body with cold water you'll force the lymph vessels to contract, helping to flush lymph fluid and push that unwanted waste out of your body.

#6 Quicker recovery from your workouts

Many top class sports stars these days use ice baths. It's widely known that this exposure to extreme cold helps soothe the muscles and bring down swelling and soreness.

You don't have to go right to that extreme as cold showers can have a significant effect in fighting those inflammatory markers, as well as removing lactic acid from your muscles more quickly.

#7 Energy rush

Nothing will wake you up like a cold shower does. And there's little that will leave you feeling as alert and energized when you step out of that shower.

This links back to the boost of neurotransmitters in the brain, and stimulation of your endocrine system, by the blast of cold water, as referred to earlier.

Want to feel fired up for the day ahead? Then forget the hot, opt for the cold instead.

Warming Up For The Cold Approach

The idea of taking a full 5 minute cold shower is probably a horrendous prospect to you right now. I get it. But if you're new to this, it's a much better idea to ease yourself into it and gradually adapt.

Here's what I suggest...

Stage 1

- Taking a warm shower as normal and then begin by turning the setting to cold for the last 20 seconds only. Do this each day for a full week.

Stage 2

- Do the same as above, but increase the time under cold water to 45-60 secs. Do this for another week.

Stage 3

- Cold shower from the beginning and, if need be, adapt to the cold in stages. i.e. run your left arm under the water for 5 secs, then your right arm for 5 secs, then your chest, then the crown of your head, face, and when you finally feel brave enough...flip round to your back.

(Optional): let out a high-pitched sissy scream if no-one else is at home.

CHAPTER 16

Health Hacking Through 'Hoffing'

Growing up as a kid in the 80s, I had three sets of heroes...

The A-Team, Thundercats, and The Hoff. The latter being David Hasselhoff of course, who starred as Michael Knight in one of my favourite TV programmes 'Knightrider'.

But I gradually went off The Hoff. He switched from Knightrider to Baywatch, swapping his black leather jacket and talking sports car for skimpy red shorts and running along a beach in slow motion.

His coolness instantly dropped by around 10% in my eyes. Then The Hoff released some cheesy - and slightly creepy – song inviting you to 'jump into his car' that definitely brought him down another few notches in the cool famous people stakes.

Last year, The Hoff began starring in super cringey adverts in the UK for a frozen food store. It was then well and truly time to pull the ejector seat on my Knightrider childhood hero. Partly because I'm now a 36-year-old man.

But when one door closes on a Hoff, another opens to welcome a brand new, much cooler HOF.

This Hof also walks about bare-chested and bare-footed, but forget sandy beaches...he treks up Mount Everest and Kilimanjaro instead.

This Hof also dives into water regularly in his shorts, but forget American surfing in the sunshine...he breaks through frozen-over lakes and goes for long swims under the ice.

And while the mega uncool David Hasselhoff releases cheesy music records, cool-as-ice Wim Hof is busy setting new world records. He's got nearly 20 in the bag already.

You may well already have heard of the incredible human that is Wim Hof. And if this is your first introduction to The Iceman, then it was only a matter of time before you came across him.

The 59-year-old wacky Dutchman is fast becoming a global icon and his Wim Hof Method is amassing more and more followers across the world every day.

Why? Because Wim Hof has disproved what scientists have long thought wasn't possible: that we can control our autonomic nervous system, immune system, and endocrine system to take charge of our health, happiness and strength.

Wim Hof says it's all possible through the three pillars of his ground-breaking method: cold therapy, breathing technique, and concentration and mindset development.

There are now scientific papers that back Wim's method up because he underwent numerous tests to prove his bold claim that he could control his autonomic, nervous and immune systems.

Then when skeptics concluded that he must be a freak of nature, Hof trained a dozen ordinary people to do the same in just two weeks. The results were mind-blowing.

There are countless stories of people across the world using the Wim Hof Method to help reverse long-standing health conditions such as fibromyalgia, speed up recovery from injuries, and even beat depression.

These remarkable tales are all over the web in blogs, videos, and discussed regularly in the Wim Hof Method Facebook group, which has over 110,000 members at the time of writing this in early 2019. I've included a couple of examples in the bibliography/reference section at the end of this book.

The reason the Wim Hof Method is so effective? The cold therapy combined with the special breathing technique drastically reduces inflammation levels in the body.

I strongly believe the Wim Hof Method is one of the most powerful natural health hacks. It'll help you recover properly and more quickly from tough workouts. It'll help boost your immune system so you can stay strong and healthy. It'll keep your mind sharp, alert and reduce any anxiety/depressive symptoms.

I'm going to briefly describe the Wim Hof Method, the science behind it, and explain how I've easily applied 'Hoffing' to my own daily routine. But I'm not an expert and I'd highly recommended learning from the main man himself.

Wim Hof has created a free, short video course where you can learn the fundamentals of his method at: https://www.wimhofmethod.com/free-mini-class

It's split into three lessons – 'The Power Of Breathing', 'The Power Of Cold Showers', and 'The Power Of Your Mind' – which are all well worth watching. I'm a huge Hof fan, and I reckon you'll become one too.

A Simple Health Hack In 15 Mins Per Day

My daily Wim Hof Method routine simply involves a cold shower in the morning, and then once I'm dressed I do the breathing technique for around 15 mins.

We've already covered braving cold showers in the previous chapter, but the breathing technique will likely be new to you.

The main purpose of the breathing technique is to flood your body with extra oxygen and change the overall ratio of oxygen and carbon dioxide in your system. Oxygen is used by cells of the body's tissues, while carbon dioxide is produced as a waste product.

When your cells are short of oxygen the tissues become inflamed. Chronic inflammation, as described earlier, means your cells have been starved of oxygen. Infection can take hold and bacteria will further starve the cells of oxygen, eventually leading to disease.

Chronic stress can also have an impact on the body's oxygen levels as it affects your natural breathing rhythm. Think about what happens when we become panicked, angry or highly stressed.

People will say, "take a deep breath" and try to calm you down. That's because you're hyperventilating due to an automatic change in breathing where we take in less oxygen and there's more carbon dioxide in our system.

Even if it doesn't quite reach the hyperventilation stage, many people breathe shallow for long periods in the day either because they're working stressful jobs, or they're very unfit and carrying a lot of excess weight.

All of this leads to your body's cells receiving less oxygen, which goes hand in hand with inflammation.

The beauty of the Wim Hof breathing technique is that it lowers carbon dioxide levels and hits your body with a tidal wave of oxygen that you wouldn't otherwise get in any normal day.

Below I'll explain how it's done in three parts, but first here are a few important safety precautions:

- Don't take the Wim Hof Method and techniques too lightly. They go deep and the effects can have a huge impact.
- Never do the breathing exercises in a swimming pool, beneath the shower, while in charge of any vehicle, or any place where the risk of fainting may cause harm. Always practice the breathing exercises in a safe environment.
- Do the breathing exercises without forcing them, gradually build up and don't exceed your limits.

Part One

Take a deep intake of breath in through your mouth, and then release without forcing. Inhale very deeply again, and then let go gently once more, and so on.

The idea is that by breathing in more deeply than normal, and exhaling gently, you're positively changing the ratio between oxygen and carbon dioxide in your blood.

You repeat this form of deep inhale/gentler exhale breathing for 30 rounds.

Part Two

After the 30th exhale, stop and hold your breath for up to 2 mins. By this point the body is loaded with oxygen, but by not taking any more air into your lungs, there is a build-up of CO_2. The body compensates for this extra CO_2 by pulling more oxygen into the cells.

This is where the big benefits come. In addition, the series of deep inhalations also stimulates the endocrine system and causes the body to pump out high levels of hormones like adrenaline and noradrenaline.

This is why many people report that the Wim Hof breathing technique energizes them and some describe it as "euphoric".

Part Three

The aim is to hold your breath for up to 2 mins, but some people barely reach a minute on their first attempt. When you reach your maximum breath hold, you release, and then take in another single big inhalation of air, and hold that for 10-15 secs.

Those three parts equal one full round, and should last around 4-5 mins. Best practice is to do three rounds in quick succession, which means you'll be finished the whole practice within 15 mins.

As I mentioned earlier, I do my breathing session in the morning after coming out of a cold shower. Sometimes I'll do it again in the evening after a busy, stressful day. I also usually take an additional cold shower after my gym workouts.

The Science Behind Hoffing

The autonomic nervous system regulates the body on a subconscious level, keeping everything ticking along nicely in the background. It takes care of breathing, your heart beating, digestion, contraction of blood vessels etc.

It was previously thought that this was strictly automatic and we could not consciously control our body's autonomic nervous system. A 2011 study suggested that Wim Hof was able to influence his autonomic nervous system - and the science world began to sit up and take notice.

Researchers at Radboud University in the Netherlands set up a study involving Wim Hof and 112 other participants. Each person was injected with bacteria expected to trigger flu-like symptoms in a matter of hours.

Remarkably, Hof only experienced a mild headache when the symptoms were supposed to be at their strongest. His body also produced half the inflammatory proteins compared to the average of others in the study.

The study leader concluded that Hof was able to control his immune response to the bacteria through his concentration technique. This triggered the release of more cortisol which suppressed the inflammatory proteins – and kept the flu symptoms at bay.

A fluke? A feat only achievable by this special Dutchman? Not according to Hof, and he went onto prove anybody can yield this same power over their own body by practising the Wim Hof technique.

In 2013, Hof spent 10 days training a group of 12 Dutch men to do the same as him. They followed the breathing practice, learned meditation techniques for superior focus, and were gradually exposed to cold water conditions.

Those 12 people – and another 12 control group volunteers – were later injected with the same bacteria as Wim Hof in the previous study. The individuals who were trained in the Wim Hof Method reported much milder symptoms, such as headaches, nausea and shivers, than the control group.

Meanwhile, their body temperature also stayed closer to baseline compared to the control group. These astonishing findings were published in the scientific journal PNAS (Proceedings of the National Academy of Sciences of the USA) in 2014.

If you want to learn more about this study and the fascinating science behind the Wim Hof Method you can download a free e-book at: https://www.wimhofmethod.com/science

While I'm sure you don't intend to be injected with bacteria anytime soon, the immune-boosting potential of the Wim Hof Method could help keep you healthy and strong.

Meanwhile, the anti-inflammatory effects of cold showers and breathing technique could play a big role in your recovery from workouts, injuries, and possibly even chronic health conditions.

In the UK, where I live, these non-steroidal anti-inflammatory drugs (NSAIDs) are one of the most commonly prescribed medications.

They are also associated with more emergency hospital admissions due to adverse drug reactions than any other class of medicine, according to a British Medical Journal report published in 2018.

That's quite worrying when you consider that there are also highly effective, natural ways to reduce inflammation in the body.

Two gifts from nature: the cold and the breath.

CHAPTER 17

The Fast Lane To Recovery

Fitness is 30% exercise and 70% nutrition, said some wise health expert/mathematician.

Or were they wise, really? This phrase has been circulating around in the fitness world so long that it's basically become a cliché. We all get the thinking behind it, though: you can train like a warrior, but if your diet sucks, you won't get very far.

There's a third important element that's been left out. Something that doesn't get the attention it deserves, yet could be the difference between you reaching your fitness goals within 3 months or 3 years.

I'm talking about proper recovery. The hard work in the gym and good nutrition are just two pieces of the puzzle. To get the most from your workouts, strip fat efficiently, build muscle tissue effectively, and sculpt a stronger, healthier body, there's got to be a conscious effort to recover well.

Don't expect to get anywhere fast with your fitness goals if you're up late watching Netflix every night, boozing throughout the weekend, and not giving your body enough rest and repair time after workouts.

At the same time, over-training can halt your progress. Hitting the weights hard day after day, or doing high-intensity training most of the week, can have a detrimental effect in the long run.

I'm talking joint pain, tissue damage, and ultimately frazzling your nervous system if you're going at it too hard for too long. This can lead to running down your immune system, taxing your adrenal glands (which act like your body's battery), and ending up feeling burnt-out.

I did an interview a few years ago with renowned fitness expert Ru Anderson, founder of Exceed Nutrition. I asked for his top three tips for looking, feeling and performing at your best.

His number one tip? <u>Focus on recovery</u>.

He said: "A big factor to bigger muscles and greater strength is the ability to fully recover from your training efforts. Train hard, but ensuring you can recover from it is key.

"Many magazines and programs can push your recovery abilities too far, because they have been created by athletes - or those using assistance."

But how much training equals overtraining? Is there a maximum time in the gym, a ceiling on the number of exercises you should be doing, or ideal number of days you should be working out per week?

Short answer – no. Slightly longer answer – everybody is different, and our fitness levels, workout duration, intensity etc all influence your body's ability to recover.

This is why I always recommend a one day on, one day off training schedule when it comes to heavy weight training and/or high-intensity interval training. Just 3-4 training sessions per week is ideal.

The strain from weight training causes tiny tears on the muscle fibres, leading to inflammation and DOMS (delayed onset muscle soreness) afterwards. If you've been training hard enough you should naturally be sore the following day, and probably even sorer the next day.

That's why you need proper rest in between gym sessions. Your body takes full advantage of the down time and the nutrients from good food to properly repair these small muscle tears and overcompensate for them.

This is when the body is actually being remodelled. Not in the gym, but in the hours that follow, particularly when you're sleeping. So, it doesn't make sense to interrupt that process and working out regularly on consecutive days will only lead to overtraining and hamper your progress.

You'll increase your chances of injury. You'll increase the likelihood of becoming run-down. And you'll not achieve your health and fitness goal any sooner.

What if you're one of those workout maniacs who actually just enjoys the feel good buzz of exercising every day? I get it, sometimes I like to throw in an extra workout if I'm having a crappy day and want to de-stress.

In this case, there is a work-around. Always maintain the day's rest after a heavy weight training session, however you could do a sprint training session instead. Alternatively, you could still hit the gym but do an abs-only workout, giving your larger muscle groups a rest.

The abdominals are more resilient and take more effort to be fatigued, therefore you could focus on doing a series of abs isolation exercises such as: oblique twists, leg raises, abs rollouts, mountain climbers etc.

Essentials For Quicker Recovery From Your Workouts

Sufficient sleep

Might seem like I'm stating the obvious here, but it's important to underline that there's nothing more powerful than a proper night's sleep for recovery from your workouts, recovery from illness, and restoring balance in our often hectic lives.

You could eat the healthiest food, drink the best brand of protein shakes, take all the fancy supplements at the health food store, but if you're sleep deprived you're going to get nowhere.

You'll struggle to lose weight, you'll struggle to get rid of toxins, you'll throw your hormones out of whack and struggle to build muscle, you'll feel fatigued, your immune system will suffer, the list goes on.

When it comes to hitting your fitness goals, sleep is a major player. That's why I've dedicated the entire next chapter to properly explaining why, and helping you optimise your sleeping pattern.

More magnesium

Magnesium is sometimes referred to as the relaxation mineral. It's a critical nutrient that's responsible for the function of 325 enzyme reactions in the body and can be found in all of your tissues, but mainly in muscle, bone and the brain.

Magnesium is essential for your cells to make energy, and plays numerous other important roles in the body. Yet it's estimated that many Americans are "dangerously deficient" due to stress and bad dietary choices robbing their bodies of magnesium.

The Recommended Daily Allowance (RDA) of magnesium is between 350mg and 400mg, but Dr Carolyn Dean, author of The Magnesium Miracle, suggests that twice as much is needed for optimal health and warding off 22 conditions that are directly linked to magnesium deficiency.

As well as addressing a possible deficiency, there are several reasons why supplementing with magnesium can help you recover more effectively from a hard workout.

It relaxes the muscles and also helps lower inflammation. That's why some health experts recommend an Epsom salt (magnesium sulfate) bath for athletes or people with muscle and joint pain, swelling or sprains.

However, spraying magnesium oil onto the skin is a much better option as it'll ensure much more of this magnificent mineral is absorbed. Ancient Minerals is the brand I use, and can be bought online via the Amazon website.

Magnesium also helps calm the nervous system and regulates cortisol – a hormone released by the body in times of stress or during intense exercise. This makes it an ideal supplement to take after working out/before going to bed at night.

Extreme temperatures

From one end of the spectrum with cold showers to the other end where you sweat out it out in the sauna, extreme temperatures have been proven to help you recover better from your workouts.

I've already covered cold showers in detail and how they bring down inflammation, and thus speed up healing and recovery. Therefore, let's look more closely at the benefits of going for a sauna a couple of times per week.

I don't know about you, but I absolutely love the sauna and like to go 1-2 times per week (ideally on my rest days from the gym). There's something about becoming a hot, steaming, sweaty mess that helps me relax and unwind big time.

We all know that saunas are great for ridding your body of toxins, but the high temperatures are also effective for helping people ease the aftermath of tough workouts and assist the body in recovering more quickly.

Saunas increase circulation and raise the body's temperature, which helps fight aches, pains and relieves muscle tension. These culminate in a quicker recovery time between workouts.

Looking for an even better reason to sweat it out in the sauna? A 2015 study involving 2,315 men from Finland between the ages of 42 and 60 showed that taking a sauna 2-3 times per week reduced their risk of dying from heart attacks, heart disease, cardiovascular disease, and cancer by 27%.

Those who had a sauna 4-7 times per week reduced their risk by 50%. The detailed research was carried out over a 20 year period and showed these startling results.

Dr Rhonda Patrick PhD, a scientist and creator of Foundmyfitness.com, has done extensive research into the benefits of sauna use, as well as fasting, and exercise.

She says that the heat stress caused by saunas can also help athletes improve their endurance, prevent muscle breakdown through disuse, and improve insulin sensitivity by increasing the number of glucose receptors in the muscle cells.

It might sound a bit counter-intuitive when you're first hearing about the benefits of the extreme cold and then extreme heat. Like cold showers and hot saunas don't go together.

Oh yes they do. And there's nothing quite like leaving a wooden box fired up to 100 degrees centigrade and stepping straight into a 10 degrees cold shower.

That'll quickly waken you up. On that note, let's now dive into hacking your sleep so that you can maximise the benefits of your workouts and optimise your overall health.

CHAPTER 18

Maximise Your Workouts With Enhanced Sleep

Alan sat in the chair across the table from Rosalie mesmerised by the machine she was messing around with - and the weird noises it was making.

On the table were rows of small glass test tubes. There were dozens of them, side by side, and Rosalie was touching each one with a small steel wand.

Every now and again a high-pitched noise would sound from the 'Vega' machine that the wand was connected to. Rosalie would then take some notes, before moving onto the next test tube with the wand.

It was Alan's first visit to this alternative health place in the countryside, and it was his 100th attempt to figure out why he was always feeling run-down and fatigued.

Alan didn't know what was going on. Neither did his doctor, who just wanted to palm him off with prescription after prescription. So, going down the homeopathic route was the next option.

Playing football on Tuesdays and Fridays, Alan was always pretty active. He even did high-intensity strength and conditioning fitness classes a couple of times each week too.

Although his diet was never the greatest – Alan had a loving relationship with donner kebabs – he'd at least been making healthier food choices for a couple of months. Yet he was still feeling tired and sluggish every day.

While his doctor seemed pretty clueless about it all, Alan got a good feeling within minutes of his consultation with Rosalie. He liked the vibe of her alternative health centre, the attention being paid to him, and the different type of approach being taken.

Rosalie had been running her facility for nearly 40 years, and always had a waiting list of 3-6 months. That was a good sign, he figured. Another good sign was that she was aged in her 80s, and literally looked and behaved 30 years younger.

Alan filled in a lengthy questionnaire before sitting down for the proper consultation. The questions on the form weren't what he was expecting. One of the first was about vaccinations he'd had in his life, and when he received them. He was asked about prescribed antibiotics, the medication he was on, his diet, and more.

Rosalie put his questionnaire to one side. She'd only read it after working her magic with the wand and the Vega machine. Even without the form, this part of the consultation would give her the answers she needed.

Alan was sat in a magnetic chair that connected with the Vega machine. Rosalie was controlling the machine at the other side of the table.

Vega testing, which has its origins in acupuncture and homeothapy, isn't well known but is used to identify illness in the body. The machine measures the body's energy levels, revealing blockages and problem areas to the alternative health practitioner.

As Alan sat in the chair, Rosalie was essentially scanning his body with her unique method. The wand would touch each glass tube, which contained all sorts of vitamins and minerals. Whenever a high pitch sound was made, it meant that blockages and micronutrient deficiencies had been discovered.

Rosalie took note after note, each one like a puzzle piece in determining what was wrong with Alan. Fifteen minutes later, she had the diagnosis. Adrenal fatigue, a deficiency in B vitamins, and low levels of some minerals too.

"Do you work different shifts?" asked Rosalie.

Alan replied: "Yes, I've been working backshifts and nightshifts for years. My working hours change quite regularly."

Rosalie: "You have to get off those shifts. That's the root cause of these health problems. You're sleep-deprived and your body's circadian rhythm is all over the place.

"Proper sleep is so important."

The Vega machine also gave Alan a biological age rating, and it suggested his body was functioning like that of a man in his mid-50s. Alan was just 32 at the time.

He was urged to buy Floradix – a liquid iron and vitamins drink – to help bring his energy levels back up. Rosalie also gave Alan some other natural vitamin and minerals supplements to deal with his deficiencies.

I know this story about my friend Alan going to this alternative health place - and the use of the Vega machine - sounds a bit 'woo-woo'. It did to me at first too, until I experienced it first-hand.

Whether you believe in homeothapy or alternative health practices or not doesn't matter. I'm not trying to convince you either way.

But the results do matter.

Those supplements had my friend Alan feeling recharged within weeks. He still had energy when he was coming home later at night after his backshifts. He wasn't feeling as burnt-out the day after his nightshifts.

Still, Rosalie warned him that those working patterns and lack of sleep were the root cause of his health problems. They were shaving years off his life, and he'd been like a guy in his 50s in a 32-year-old body.

A few months later, he got a job promotion at the whisky bottling factory where he works. Better money, a more enjoyable role and, most importantly, 9-5 working hours.

He's now getting to travel to countries like India and France to meet suppliers for their whisky company, and is much healthier and happier these days.

Six months after his initial consultation, Alan returned for a follow-up with Rosalie. They went through the whole process again, but Alan already knew what the outcome was going to be. He was feeling too good for the Vega machine results to be bad.

Rosalie told him that his health was much improved, and that biological age had dropped back down to mid-30s – exactly where it should be.

"The body knows how to heal itself," she told him. "We just have to give it the right tools – and enough sleep is the most important one."

Your Muscles Grow In Bed, Not The Gym

The hard work is done in the gym, but the development of your muscles and reshaping of your body happens when you're snoozing. Sleep enhances muscle recovery through protein synthesis and the release of anabolic hormones.

If you want to build more muscle, become leaner, and improve your overall body shape, then stop messing around – and get to your bed!

Exercise is a form of stress to the body, and weight training in particular leads to tears in your muscle fibres and can cause a strain on your joints. Your sleeping hours are when the body goes to work on the repair and rebuilding process.

Naturally, the tougher the training session the more time it's going to take to rebuild the body – and therefore the more sleep you require. Five, six, and sometimes even seven, is not going to cut it.

Most adults aged 18-64 need 7-9 hours of sleep per night, according to experts at the National Sleep Foundation. But athletes and people like you pushing your body extremely hard in your workouts may need that little bit more.

Sleep is crucial to the muscle recovery process because this is when there are spurts of anabolic hormones, which are central to muscle development and fat breakdown.

When you go to bed your body is primed to produce increased amounts of anabolic hormones, such as IGF-1, growth hormone, and testosterone, while the level of catabolic hormones is reduced. The delivery of nutrients to your muscles in also enhanced.

Studies have shown that spikes of growth hormone occur when you're sleeping between 10pm and 2am. So you can see why staying up late watching reality TV, or wasting time on Facebook at night doesn't just melt your brain, it interferes with your body's ability to develop muscle and remodel itself after a workout.

The 24-Hour Circadian Rhythm And Stages Of Sleep

I don't want to put you to sleep on sleep, but it's useful to understand the body's natural circadian rhythm, and the different stages of sleep.

A circadian rhythm is a 24-hour cycle managed by our body clock. This clock is located within your brain and is in control of your internal systems such as your hormone production, body temperature, sleeping and eating patterns, mood and alertness.

Your body clock is set by external factors such as daylight, temperature and meal times. During the circadian rhythm there are a number of changes in your body's hormone production.

For example, at sunrise the light receptors in our eyes and on our skin are stimulated. These are part of the central nervous system and they signal to the brain that it's time to wake up and start the day.

The receptors also message the brain to release cortisol, which makes us alert and ready for the day ahead. Cortisol drops to a low level by lunchtime, and by sundown hits its lowest levels.

Sundown also triggers the release of melatonin, the hormone which helps regulate our sleep, and this has a knock-on effect of triggering the release of other hormones such as testosterone, estrogen, and growth hormone.

Sleep ain't just any old sleep. There are five stages of sleep that are repeated in a cycle several times during the night, but we can simplify matters by breaking them into two main stages: deep sleep and REM (rapid eye movement) sleep.

Deep sleep is essential for muscle recovery and restoring the body. During this phase your blood pressure drops and your breathing becomes slower and deeper. It accounts for around 40% of your total sleep time.

As your brain is resting with little activity, the blood supply to your muscles increases, delivering extra oxygen and nutrients for growth and healing. This is when muscle tissue damaged during your workouts is repaired and remodelled.

This deep sleep phase is also when your pituitary gland releases growth hormone to facilitate that muscle growth and repair. A lack of sleep causes a significant drop in growth hormone production.

REM sleep happens in cycles of 90-120 minutes and dominates the later hours just before waking. This stage of sleep provides energy to the brain and this is when the brain becomes more active, slipping into a dreams phase. REM sleep helps restore the mind for the day ahead.

As you can see, the deep sleep part deals primarily with restoring and repairing your body, while the latter REM phase is focused more on psychological processing and recovery.

What The Sleep Experts Say

In her book *The Business of Sleep*, Professor Vicki Culpin, a clinical psychologist and sleep expert, warns: "Never before have significant percentages of working adults been so sleep deprived."

Her book describes "an age of foolishness" in which many people seem unaware of the "serious cognitive and health consequences" of insufficient or poor quality sleep.

Professor Culpin warns that anyone who gets less than seven hours rest a night is at heightened risk of damage to their physical or mental health. A 2013 study by the National Sleep Foundation involving six countries – America, the UK, Germany, Japan, Canada and Mexico – found that people are regularly falling short.

Researchers conducted telephone interviews with a total of 1,500 people from these countries and found two thirds of Japanese people (66%) say they sleep less than seven hours on work nights.

This is compared to 53% of the Americans, 39% of UK residents, 36% of Germans, 30% of Canadians and 29% of Mexicans. Meanwhile, one in five Americans (21%), Japanese (19%) and people in the UK (18%) reported sleeping less than six hours a night during the work week.

In 2018, Professor Culpin gave a fascinating Ted Talk titled 'A Wake Up Call: This Talk Should Send You To Sleep'.

She told the audience: "Poor sleep is endemic across the world and we know so much now about the impact of it. At any point in time, if you are consistently sleeping for less than six hours a night, your risk of dying increases by 13%. Between 6 and 7 hours, it still increases your mortality risk by 7%.

"You're 3-4 times more likely to get cold and flu. You're more likely to get some types of cancer, particularly if you do shift work over long periods of time."

Tips For Getting A Better Night's Sleep

Get on a regular sleep schedule.

Go to bed and get up at the same time every day. As I mentioned earlier, the ideal time for nodding off is 10pm-10.30pm so you can make the most of the deep sleep hours and optimise anabolic hormone production.

Switch off the TV earlier – and switch off to social media.

The bright lights from the TV, mobile phone, tablets, laptops and the continued mental stimulation they cause at night interfere with your body's natural circadian rhythm. In the evening your body naturally releases melatonin - a hormone that helps regulate our sleep.

Studies have shown that every hour you're still on your mobile phone/tablet/laptop/watching TV at night, melatonin is suppressed by 30 minutes. This digital world we're living in is messing with nature, it's messing with our natural circadian rhythm, and it's messing with our hormones.

If you still need to use your digital device late at night, perhaps for reading on your mobile phone or laptop, you can adjust the colour and reduce the amount of blue light with software such as f.lux or by using Apple's Night Shift mode.

Create a sleep-friendly environment

Considering you spend roughly a third of your life in bed, it's worth investing in a good quality bed frame, mattress and comfortable pillows.

If too much light gets into the room, why not use a black-out blind or curtains? Turn the power off on the TV or other digital devices to wipe out distracting flashing lights. Put your mobile phone on silent before putting your head down on the pillow, or turn it off completely and use an old-fashioned alarm clock.

Exercise in the morning

There are long-standing 'sleep hygiene' tips that recommend not exercising too close to bedtime. Some health experts believe that the rush of adrenaline and extra stimulation of the nervous system may cause difficulty in nodding off, while other sleep experts argue that any exercise is better than no activity at all for sleep.

But an interesting study was carried out with 14 athletes in 2018 to determine the effects of morning exercise on sleep compared to evening exercise. They looked closely at moderate and vigorous exercise intensities for both times in the day.

The researchers concluded: "Higher sleep efficiency was found when the training is performed in the morning compared to the evening sessions in both intensities."

A 7am gym session, doing a 30 mins super sets workout, surely isn't out of the question? Of course, this all depends on your work commitments or parenting duties, and you'll have to factor in whether or not you're a morning or night person. More on that in the next chapter.

Stick With The Programme

Don't skip workouts. Being consistent with your weekly training regime will have a positive impact on your sleep quality – and vice versa.

Vigorous exercisers are almost twice as likely as non-exercisers to sleep well every night or almost every night during the week. They also are the least likely to report sleep problems.

That is according to the National Sleep Foundation 2013 Poll, which surveyed 1,000 people in America to determine the relationship between exercise and sleep.

More than two-thirds of vigorous exercisers said they rarely or never (in the previous two weeks) had symptoms commonly associated with insomnia, including waking up too early and not being able to get back to sleep

The study also concluded that all exercisers - vigorous, moderate and light - are significantly more likely to say "I had a good night's sleep" every night or almost every night on work nights than people who don't work out.

Avoid sleep medication.

Unless a doctor has prescribed it, don't take any sleep medications. Over-the-counter sleep aids are likely to disturb the quality of your sleep and your performance the next day.

Relying on natural relaxation techniques before bed - such as deep breathing or meditation - is a better approach. Natural supplements, such as magnesium oil or ZMA (zinc, magnesium, vitamin B6 formulation) tablets, will not only help you nod off, but they'll give your body a helping hand for repair and development.

Cut back on alcohol and caffeine.

I'm stating the obvious here when it comes to caffeine as I'm sure you're well aware that it's a stimulant. Too many cups of coffee and you're wired. A couple of energy drinks and you're tuned to the moon.

At the same time, I know lots of people can't function without coffee in the morning and during their work day. Here's a smart move: simply stop drinking tea or coffee by 3pm. This will give your body time to get the caffeine out of your system and your nervous system time to chill the hell out.

It's estimated that around 20% of Americans use alcohol to help them get to sleep. A glass of wine or two in the evening, or stopping off at the pub after working late.

It turns out that boozing actually has the opposite effect as it affects the quality of your sleep and, over time, it can lead to insomnia. This is because alcohol disrupts your body's natural circadian rhythm.

Researchers from the University of Missouri School of Medicine in the US have studied the relationship between alcohol consumption and sleep for over five years.

They reported that alcohol disrupts sleep, the quality of sleep is diminished, and the fact that it's a diuretic means that it increases your need to go to the toilet during the night and earlier in the morning.

If you want to maximise the results from your hard-earned workouts, it's time for some hardcore sleeping!

Switch off the lights, and I'll see you in the next chapter.

BONUS INTERVIEW

With Elite Sports Sleep Coach Nick Littlehales

"Yes, it's a given that a healthy adult needs around eight hours of recovery in every 24. Nobody is arguing with that. But how you get it can be different."

That final sentence got stuck in my brain when I chatted with Nick Littlehales at length about the brain and sleep. It was late on a Tuesday afternoon and we were supposed to be having a quick 15-minute telephone conversation about sleep and recovery.

Those 15 minutes turned into 94 as the renowned sleep expert blew my brain to pieces with his knowledge and advice on proper recovery. I soaked up every second of this golden information and by the end of the phone call I knew that my daily approach to sleep would be changed forever.

By the end of this chapter yours might well be too.

If you're someone who has always struggled with sleep, work a stressful job, and want to recover properly – but just can't – then Nick's unique approach to sleep and recovery could be a complete game-changer for you.

Nick Littlehales has become known as 'The Elite Sports Sleep Coach'...the guy who helps the biggest sports stars around the world get a better quality of shut eye every day.

Nick's fascinating approach, known as the R90 Human Recovery Technique, is so effective that the Englishman has worked with some of the most famous sporting names on the planet including leading European Premiership and Championship clubs, such as Manchester City, Real Madrid, Liverpool, Manchester United, Norwich City, Brentford, Cardiff City and Brighton and Hove Albion.

He's also worked with the England national football team, supported British Cycling and Team Sky at the London 2012 Olympics, the Netherlands bobsleigh team before the 2014 Winter Olympics, American NFL and NBA teams, a host of athletes at the 2016 Olympic Games in Rio, and onto the Tokyo 2020 Olympics where he'll be supporting athletes in all sports from netball and snowboarding to equestrian riders and BMX stars.

Sporting coaches and organisations, who always took exercise and nutrition so seriously, recognised the huge impact sleep quality has on performance, health and wellbeing that they drafted in Nick and his team for a professional approach to recovery.

The Sports Sleep Coach role was born in 1996 when Sir Alex Ferguson, who was manager of Manchester United FC at the time, called upon Nick's expertise. Nick had been international sales and marketing director of Slumberland, the largest sleeping comfort group in Europe in the late 90s.

Around the same time, sports science was limited but the importance of recovery was being recognised. Sir Alex called in Nick, and soon the Manchester United players, manager and even the coaching staff were following Nick's sleep strategies, and using his products to perform at their best each week.

These days Nick talks to athletes about their daily habits, gives them advice and a strategy to manage their rest in cycles. He designs and sources their sleeping products, and helps them create the best sleeping environments at home and on their travels.

When I spoke with Nick I had my list of questions written out in front of me, voice recorder at the ready, and writing pad for taking some back-up notes in shorthand in case the recording somehow failed.

Having worked as a journalist for 15 years in my previous life, I was always well prepared for interviews. But this call with Nick didn't exactly go to plan.

After first asking "what are your top five tips for to help anyone get a better night's sleep?", the conversation quickly took a different direction.

"Right....well, it's not quite the top tips that you read about all the time. 'Don't eat too late, sort your bedroom out, shut your tech down'...all these pieces of advice that are generic and have been around for years," said Nick.

"In my long career in the sleep industry, and in the last 22 years in sport, a lot has changed since the 90s.

"We started getting phones, computers, all these digital devices, and the dynamics inside of sport has also changed. There's an international commitment of athletes, dealing with the media, and just about everyone else has a camera.

"We've had to redefine sleep and start talking about physical and mental recovery because the word 'sleep' puts us in a place of something we take for granted.

"We try to get this myth of eight hours per night. Nobody achieves it, and we're not doing anything about it. It's time to start talking about sleep differently, without losing what it's about.

"What sleep is really about is physical and mental recovery."

Mental And Physical Recovery...In Cycles

Sleep in today's digital world is a completely different ball game from that of our ancestors. Our brains are wired with all the constant activity. Our natural circadian rhythm is out of whack. We want eight hours per night - but we don't know how.

Surely there must be another way? There is, according to Nick.

The first step is redefining sleep as physical and mental recovery.

The second is to achieve the required amount of physical and mental recovery in a different way.

That means switching from our normal 'monophasic' (once in 24 hours) way of sleeping to 'polyphasic', which means several times in any given day (aka introducing naps).

"Humans have always slept in a polyphasic manner," said Nick. "We only started sleeping monophasically when we invented electric light."

At the core of what Nick teaches people all over the world is switching back to that polyphasic way of sleeping, and it's particularly effective for achieving the required rest in today's busy modern world.

While most of us struggle to get eight hours in one go per night, sleeping polyphasically helps us get sufficient rest in chunks over the course of 24 hours.

But there's much more to it than that. There are several other key factors to achieving the mental and physical recovery Nick talks about so that you can look, feel and perform at your best each day.

These include:

- Sleeping in 90-minute recovery cycles, rather than 8-hour periods, and aiming for 35 cycles per week.
- Learning about circadian rhythms and living in harmony with them.
- Introducing CRPs (controlled recovery periods) – naps and activity breaks (i.e. taking breaks from your work desk, a relaxing walk in daylight outside etc to ease stress and the strain on your brain).
- Adopting a balanced approach to recovery and activity throughout the day, again to support your brain function...and making it easier for you to sleep at night.
- Easing into your day in the morning, with hydration, exposure to natural sunlight, and gentle mental challenges etc, as your first daily recovery period.
- Optimising your post-sleep routine, NOT your pre-sleep routine as most people do.
- Changing your perception of your bedroom from your 'private sanctuary' or 'boudoir' to your mental and physical recovery room.

- Changing your bedroom environment to remove things that can become psychological barriers to sleep.
- Sleeping in the ideal position – which is the foetal position on your non-dominant side.

We'll delve into all of these below as Nick talks about his seven key sleep recovery indicators, R90 KSRIs. He insists that each of these R90 KSRIs add up to transformative results when it comes to sleep, performance, health and wellbeing.

Nick's R90 Technique – recovery in 90-minute cycles – is number three on that list. Let's now go over all of them below. I'll give a brief explanation of each, and include some supporting quotes from Nick as he elaborates further.

7 Keys To Maximising Physical And Mental Recovery

#1 Educate yourself on circadian rhythms

Circadian rhythms. Sunrise, sundown, and your internal 24-hour clock being regulated by it.

Nick: "Look at some images online of circadian rhythms of the day, and it'll clearly show you that you're just a brain with bodily functions aligned to that process. Outside, the sun is going around our planet creating light, dark and temperature shifts.

"It does it all the time, in its way, and we are completely synchronised with that. By doing a little research you'll get a clearer idea of what your body and brain wants to do when you wake up in the morning, throughout the day, what sunrise and sundown is all about, and just how much light exposure is required, when, why and at what quality."

#2 Figure out your chronotype – are you a morning or evening person?

Your chronotype describes your natural sleeping characteristics – whether you're a morning or evening person. If you're a morning person your body clock is triggered by sunrise a bit faster, while if you're the evening type there is a natural hormone phase delay of 1- 2 hours.

Nick: "The morning chronotype is affected by the sun-up process. We produce serotonin in the pineal gland as the sun comes up and the blue light comes in from the sun. Light receptors through eyelids begin to make serotonin and the brain gets the message to become active.

"The PM person/evening chronotype has a delay of 1-2 hours. They're not producing that hormone as quickly. They would prefer not to be active in the morning period, they come to life in the evening period. They have a slight phase delay relationship with melatonin and serotonin.

"You don't have to go through any scientific process to figure out your chronotype. If you have complete control over every day, when do you normally wake?

"You can camouflage it, you can adapt round it, but it's actually genetic.

"Up to 70% of the population are night-time chronotypes. Yet, up until the 90s, we very much lived in an AM-driven world. Get to work for 9am, get the kids to school, do this, do that...but things are developing a little differently these days with a 24/7 culture.

"If you don't relate to your chronotype, and don't try to manage when you do things, what you do, and why, then you may have to plan in advance to help protect you."

Some people struggle to manage their evening chronotype with cup after cup of coffee for the caffeine rush, or other unhealthy stimulants. A better option is using natural light lamps, which simulate daylight, and will speed up your body clock to get you started for the day ahead.

#3 Forget 8 hours, measure your sleep in 90-minute cycles instead

One natural sleep cycle last around 90 minutes, during which we move through 4-5 stages of sleep. When medics analyse sleeping patterns or measure brainwaves, they look at it in those 90-minute cycles.

This is why Nick recommends that we connect with our circadian rhythms, our natural sleeping cycles, and measure our recovery in these cycles rather than hours. That means breaking the 24-hour clock down into 16 segments.

The aim is to fit in 5 x 90-minute recovery cycles in over the course of the entire day, and 35 cycles over the course of any given week. On the nights where you don't sleep so well, you can compensate with controlled recovery periods, such as 30-minute power naps in the afternoon and/or early evening.

But these controlled recovery periods during the daytime don't necessarily need to be physical sleep. Breaks from your work computer screen, short relaxing walks in daylight, or a simple tea break away from your desk, can also support your daily recovery.

The focus is always on supporting your brain, and finding balance between activity and recovery.

Nick: "Five 90 mins cycles is 7.5 hours – and that's where the eight hours per night comes from.

"So, if you've got a wake time of 6am, and have five cycles of 90 mins, then you'd go back in 90 min periods to find your optimal sleep time. In this case of 6am it would be going to sleep at 10.30pm.

"We've always slept in a polyphasic manner. We only started sleeping monophasically when we invented electric light.

"So, it would be perfectly normal for you to sleep maybe three or four cycles nocturnally, wake at the consistent wake time of 6am, but also take a recovery nap of around 30 mins, either midday or evening.

"The first 90 minutes of your day should also be your first recovery break of the day. That's when you go to the toilet, when you hydrate, when you expose yourself to the light outside, and have gentle mental challenges to get your brain fully awake for the day ahead.

"So, if you're a morning person and you start to think polyphasically, you'll maximise the first part of your day and then use a little CRP to help you when you know you've got something intense to do later in the afternoon.

"Or you could use an early evening CRP to protect yourself from going to bed too early if it's summertime, the sun is still out, and you want to be proactive.

"It's all about shifting those recovery periods so you can still get enough overall sleep in a 24-hour period."

#4 The emphasis must be on your post-sleep – NOT pre-sleep – routine.

There are countless ways we try to guarantee a good sleep at night, such as not eating too late, spraying lavender fragrances on our pillows, or taking sleeping aid pills.

Most of the time it doesn't work because our brains are too wired from our busy, stressful lives – and have not been getting enough TLC throughout the day (i.e. exposure to natural sunlight, a break from mobile phone and computer screens etc).

By doing what you can to reduce stress, anxiety, get access to natural sunlight, and give your brain consistent periods of recovery from this 24/7 digital world throughout the course of the entire day, then you're going to help it switch off at night. The result...you get a better, more restful night's sleep.

Nick: "Pre-sleep is nothing more than moving from warm to cool, from light to dark. Post-sleep is about moving from cool to warm and from dark to light.

"Shutting your tech down before sleep or not eating too late, or meditating, taking supplements, listening to whale noises or whatever...is too late.

"You've got to have been doing something throughout the day that helps your brain synchronise with natural circadian rhythms.

"When you present yourself for sleep for 5 cycles, 4 cycles, 3 cycles, or little 30 mins cycles earlier in the day or early evening, the quality of sleep is down to your brain giving you what it can.

"If you get up in the morning, get exposure to natural light from outside, have a first recovery period, get on with your day, use controlled recovery periods, helping the brain as much as you can…then when you next present yourself for a long period of sleep it's going to give you the best it can.

"Because there's no such thing as a perfect night's sleep. There are so many variables in any 24 hours that are out of our control.

"What you're trying to do is use a technique that, in any 24 hours, is practical and you can have confidence in it. So, when you do ask your brain to give you some recovery at night it'll give you the best sleep possible."

#5 Have a balanced approach to activity and recovery

It's no wonder we struggle to sleep when our brains are go, go, go all day processing information from TVs, newspapers, Facebook, YouTube, emails, constant notifications on our mobile phones, the list goes on.

It never used to be that way. And we never used to have so many people in society that were sleep deprived.

Nick: "This generation just doesn't know what it's like not to have something to do. Back in the late 90s, people like me at 58 years of age now, we were travelling around the world doing very high-intensity jobs.

"But there were lots of recovery breaks because we didn't have anything to do. I could work on a plane with a pen and paper, draw graphs, take notes etc, but I couldn't do anything with it until I got to the hotel.

"We need to have a better balance between activity and recovery. That's what the R90 technique does. What you do in the first 90 minutes of your day is about recovery, as well as activity.

"Every 90 mins is about taking breaks. Take the water off your work desk and put it in the kitchen so you have to leave your desk and go walk to fetch it. It's helping the brain.

"Grab moments outside in fresh air because the light outside lights your brain up. Or use light therapy tools because we can't always be outside."

#6 Stop thinking about your bedroom as your private sanctuary or boudoir

Nick: "It's a mental and physical recovery room. It doesn't matter if you live in an apartment in a city, you share a house with a load of students, or you've got a lovely house out in the sticks. It doesn't matter if you live in Finland, Nigeria, or the west coast of America.

"When you go into your bedroom the only thing you should be worried about is that when you present yourself to sleep all you need to do is move from light to dark, and move from warm to cool.

"You'll also need the least number of stimulants in that room as possible. You'll need to be able to black it out so you can protect yourself from the seasonal changes outside, ambient light, and you'll want to be able to curl up on your mattress in the foetal position on the opposite side to your dominant side.

"The brain loves this because when humans used to sleep outside it freed up the dominant side to protect you. Your non-dominant side is also less sensitive.

"With all of that, your brain will give you the best sleep that it can. Beyond that, other people in the room like regular sleeping partners, TVs, standby lights, noise, a bed that's too small, a mattress that's too hard that won't allow you to sleep in that foetal position without a pillow, these have a negative effect.

"You might think a bedroom is a great place to watch TV, do some work, go on the laptop, spoon or cuddle with your partner, but that means you've got so many barriers to sleep in front of you.

"Your brain will not allow you to go into the deeper sleep stages if you've got all those factors involved.

"Mentally, take everything out of your bedroom. You came into the world sleeping polyphasically – fact. More sleeping periods, more often. Your parents were in a monophasic pattern and got you into a monophasic approach as soon as possible.

"You should have been sleeping polyphasically ever since you came into the world. But you've just developed a new pattern as you've got older.

"The brain has not changed. It's extremely sensitive when sleeping outside. We wouldn't sleep for long periods because it was too dangerous. We wouldn't sleep for too long because it was on a hard, uncomfortable floor.

"What we're trying to encourage people with these seven steps is that you can sleep any time, anywhere. You can sleep in a polyphasic way. You can recover in this different way.

"The daytime CRPs and naps, where you're balancing recovery with activity throughout the day, are good for your brain.

"They're creating little moments for you that cut poor perspectives – so that when you get round to an environment where you want to have a longer sleep, like nocturnally, your brain thanks you and gives you good quality sleep."

#7 The sleep kit – choosing the right products

The super mattress in the shop window might carry an extra 500 springs, along with the most expensive price tag, but that doesn't mean it's the best one for you.

Huge fluffy pillows made with duck feathers might feel nice when you first lay your head down on them, but there's a fair chance they'll lead to you twisting your neck. You'll also likely wake up several times a night to shuffle them around, trying to find a more comfortable position.

Nick isn't a fan of pillows. He's also not a fan of the one-size-fits-all approach to mattresses. He insists that our body profile types – ectomorph, mesomorph and endomorph – must be taken into consideration if we want to get the best sleep.

Using fabric layers instead of pillows are also the key to supporting the perfect sleeping position – foetal, and on your non-dominant side.

Nick: "When we come into the world, we just curl up into the foetal position and go to sleep in a cot. No pillows or anything fancy. Foetal position, on the opposite side to your dominant side, your brain likes that position.

"Why do we have a pillow? When we go on our front, we try to shift it to one side to get rid of it because our neck is twisted, or vertebrae is twisted.

"We go on our back, put the pillow behind our head and raise the neck vertebrae. It blocks the airways off, so we've got snorting, mouth breathing, and a dry mouth.

"Then when we go back into the foetal position, we start looking for the pillow to fill the gap between our head and the mattress. Why can't we have a surface that doesn't require a pillow?

"We do it with nice, soft materials. You're curled up in the foetal position, your head is touching the nice layers underneath you, there's no pillow getting in the way, and you've got more chance of going through those 90-minute cycles in deeper sleep stages.

"It's not about how much you spend in the shop. I can build you something you can sleep in the foetal position, on the opposite side to your non-dominant side, for less than £2.

"It's a bit like paying a lot of money for a personal trainer, who is coaching you running on a treadmill, but on your feet is a pair of wellington boots.

"He doesn't say to you, 'that's the wrong footwear', and trying to run in those wellington boots is going to hurt you.

"It's the same with the marketplace. Sometimes you go into the marketplace and can end up buying things that make things worse. But if you go to my website, sportsleepcoach.com, we can sort it all out for you."

Have We Forgotten The Third Pillar Of Health And Wellbeing?

The plus-side of this digital world I've been slating in this chapter is the fact that we're now more educated than ever. An answer to virtually any question is seconds away on Google. A how-to video is available through a search on YouTube. You can download millions of books to your Kindle or smartphone.

We're clued up to the max on exercise. We know far more about nutrition than we probably need to, and many of us have got a healthy obsession with health and fitness.

Nick said: "Why is it that this generation has personal trainers, we know all about nutrition beyond belief, we have so much more knowledge about how we exercise, a healthy lifestyle, we've got mindfulness, and we've got meditation?

"We've got a gym on every street corner, we know what's good for us, what's bad for us...why is it then that we've got some of the most significant increases in human mental health issues right now?

"There are three pillars of a human's health and wellbeing: eat, drink and sleep. Is it because of problems with the third pillar? We don't even chat about this, we don't educate people on it, we just don't do anything about it.

"Have we got our 5-a-day (five sleep cycles)? Not the vast majority of people.

"We go to our doctor every now and again, and invest our time speaking to them because we're concerned about our health. We get advice from personal trainers to make sure we're exercising properly.

"We buy books on nutrition and cooking, we gather information and make investments in our health and wellbeing, and in our lifestyle choices, or things we might be concerned about.

"Nobody invests in sleep – at all. All you have to do is have a conversation with someone like me. Pick the phone up, send an email, or read a book. Do it, because taking those steps can have a huge positive impact on your sleep, health and wellbeing."

RESOURCES

- Nick's book *Sleep: The Myth Of 8 Hours, The Power Of Naps, And The New Plan To Recharge Your Body and Mind - https://www.amazon.com/dp/0738234621* can be bought on the Amazon website.

- You can learn more about the R90 Technique - and book a sleep coaching call directly with Nick via his website at: https://www.sportsleepcoach.com/

MINDSET MASTERY

CHAPTER 19

Find Your Teachers

I picked up my mobile phone while still half sleeping and the first message to greet me was: "NO LIES!"

It was 5.45am. It was my first communication with any other human on a cold November morning, and it caught me off guard.

Not "good morning darling, did you have a nice sleep?" Not "do you want a cup of tea?" or any other of the other nice shit you expect to hear when you fall out of the right side of bed.

"NO LIES!" stared back at me on the screen, and it took a couple of seconds before it properly sank in. Then I nearly pissed myself laughing. It was my mate Jonathan and this was his way of giving me a swift kick up the ass to get ready for our early workout.

I didn't need it. I never need to be motivated for workouts. Whether it's lifting weights at the gym or an early morning sprints session in the rain, I've drilled it that many times that it's just a normal part of my routine, like brushing my teeth or taking a shower.

But with Jonathan, the student had become the teacher. That's what was making me laugh.

He was trying to lose weight - and I'd been trying to instill some discipline with him. Get up before 6am. Get rid of social media, emails, the news, or any other distracting and unimportant stuff. Get your ass into gear for the perfect start to any day...a tough morning workout.

"All the small things matter," I'd previously told him. "Skipping an exercise or two in the gym, drinking the bottle of cola instead of water, hitting snooze on your alarm a dozen times...they all add up. You've got to be more disciplined if you want to lose the weight and feel great."

I was acting like the PT/drill sergeant/teacher all rolled into one. Then I'd sent him a link to a video by one of my teachers – Jocko Willink. He's an ex-Navy seal war hero, who has his own podcast, has written books, and is one of the most badass badasses walking the planet today.

Jocko's motto – which is also the title of his best book – is "discipline equals freedom".

And the Jocko YouTube video I'd sent Jonathan was called "All Your Excuses Are Lies". In the three-minute clip, Jocko dishes out a no-nonsense, hardline lecture in proper drill sergeant fashion.

"The chronic excuse maker…" said Jocko in his intolerant, condescending tone. "How do you stop making excuses?

"This is actually pretty simple. You have to realise. You have to know. You have to accept…that all your excuses are LIES. They are lies – all of them."

I didn't want to keep giving Jonathan a pep talk to get himself prepared for our tough early morning workouts. I didn't want to lecture him about slacking off or making excuses. So, I let Jocko do it for me by sending that clip.

Jocko's message had clearly sunk in because Jonathan met me at Balloch Park, Loch Lomond, at 6am sharp that morning. It was cold. It was pitch black. It was hardly ideal conditions for doing hill sprints.

But we put on our woolly hats, lit up the park with two industrial lights Jonathan had swiped from his work, and began charging up that hill as fast as we could. Any early morning dog walkers who'd seen us that morning would have thought we were a couple of headcases.

It turned out to be a great session, and one of the best sprint training workouts we've ever had. We still have a laugh about it to this day, talking about the "NO LIES" text message and lighting up the pitch-black public park with our own mobile lights system.

The whole point I'm making: we all need to find our teachers.

This world has created some special, unique, inspirational characters. People who have made the impossible possible. Individuals who have overcome some incredibly tough situations in life which have helped mould them into elite figures we admire and aspire to be like.

There are not too many really special ones, but they're out there – and they're worth following to help you shape the very best version of yourself. You don't have to reinvent the wheel or spend your lifetime making a million mistakes on your road to greatness...find your teachers and take the shortcut.

That's why I consider a simple paperback book so valuable, and I think we should all read as many books as we can. Because experts condense their life's work into a book.

They include all the many things that went right in their decades' worth of experience, exclude the countless errors along the way, mention the mistakes you do need to avoid, and basically lay a roadmap for success in a particular area.

It doesn't mean it's easy when you're just starting out like a student, but with a teacher to follow you'll develop the skills more quickly, you'll start hitting goals you didn't think you had in you, and bit-by-bit you'll gradually bolt onto you the same qualities that you admired these teachers for in the first place.

Do you struggle with a positive mindset? Are you a 'chronic excuse maker', as Jocko Willink describes it? Are you simply not where you want to be fitness-wise, health-wise, financially, or in your job?

Then go out hunting for your teachers. Find five humans that are at the very top of the game you're playing. Find them – and stalk them (in a non-creepy sort of stalking way). Read their blog, buy their books, subscribe to their YouTube channels, listen to their podcast interviews, follow their Instagram page.

Absorb their knowledge every day, take it on board, and shamelessly copy them. To quote one of my top five teachers, Tony Robbins: "Long ago, I realised that success leaves clues, and that people who do outstanding results do specific things to create those results.

"I believe that if I precisely duplicated the actions of others, I could reproduce the same quality of results that they had."

I once read that a person has on average 40,000 thoughts per day. I also read that, for the average person, around 70% of those thoughts are negative. Of course, this is generalising and it's very difficult to put a number on something like this.

But our brains are wired this way to keep us safe. And there's an overload of negative drama in the world around us, from the news on the TV and the scandal in the newspapers, to the gossip in the magazines and the bitchy comments from that one particular workmate.

Too much of that garbage hurts your brain. It weakens your spirit. It affects you more than you think it does.

That's exactly why you must find your teachers and let their brilliance filter into your brain instead. Let their attitude alter yours. Let their focus and determination inspire yours. Let your mindset mirror theirs.

Switch off the news and read a teacher's book instead. Don't buy the newspaper, read a teacher's latest blog post instead. Don't bother listening to your bitchy workmate at lunchtime, go for a monster workout instead, just like one of your teachers does.

Our mindset is crafted by what we allow to filter into our mind. If you want achieve your goals in fitness, health, relationships, whatever...then what you block out is equally important as what you let in.

Here are my top 5 teachers, in no particular order: Tony Robbins, David Goggins, Jocko Willink, Jim Rohn, and Les Brown.

You've likely heard of most, if not all, of these guys because they're at the very top of their game because they've mastered their mindset. I'll give you a brief introduction to my teachers – American guys I've never met but have 'stalked' every day online for years. Then I'll share the traits I discovered they all have in common.

Tony Robbins – a one in a billion human. Tony Robbins is the guy the biggest stars in the world – Bill Clinton, Serena Williams, Hugh Jackman etc – turn to when they face the toughest challenges in their career. Suppose you could say he's the world's greatest life coach.

He's also a best-selling author and entrepreneur whose net worth in 2018 was estimated at $500 million.

David Goggins – a guy who has earned his "toughest man alive" nickname. An ex-Navy seal who has become a cult figure, particularly in the fitness world, because of his mind-blowing, record-breaking achievements.

Jocko Willink – another retired Navy Seal, who received the silver star and bronze star for his war hero efforts in Iraq. Now inspiring the masses with his no-holds barred podcasts, books, and talks.

Jim Rohn – the late entrepreneur, author and motivational speaker. Has inspired generations of successful people with his widom, and he was Tony Robbins' main teacher. Enough said.

Les Brown – entrepreneur, author, former TV host and politician, and one of the finest motivational speakers alive.

When you listen, watch and analyse these types of successful people for so long you begin to see commonalities. Strong qualities that they all share, and it doesn't take a genius to realise that these qualities are what made them so strong-minded and successful.

Discipline

This is probably the one key trait found in people who are successful and achieve their goals whether it be in fitness, their career, sports, you name it. Discipline separates the winners and the losers. It's what keeps you going when the motivation tank runs dry (and it always runs dry at some point).

If you're someone who lacks willpower when it comes to your diet, or gives into excuses too easily, then don't worry. Discipline is something you can gradually build up.

"Self-discipline is a muscle you can exercise and strengthen.

"...All disciplines affect each other. Every new discipline affects all of our other disciplines. Every new discipline that we impose on ourselves will affect the rest of our personal performance in a positive way." – Jim Rohn.

The best place to start increasing your self-discipline? Getting out of your bed earlier every morning and attacking the day. The fact that this simple discipline is your very first action of the day, it means you get the day off to a flier. It also sets you up for a more productive, positive day.

Do this every day for a week, and then stack another discipline on top of it. A cold shower in the morning? Skipping breakfast? Making a healthy power shake and holding off on drinking it until lunchtime?

You decide. Just remember that all the seemingly-small disciplines matter and stack up to big results.

They've all used adversity to their advantage

My top 5 teachers have all used the worst times in their lives to become the best versions of themselves. Rather than taking the beating from life and lying on the canvas, they've sprung back with a stronger resolve for coming through it.

Robbins was brought up by a mum who was an alcoholic and drug abuser, he had seven different stepdads, and was once completely broke.

David Goggins grew up in a house where his father regularly dished out vicious beatings to him, his mum and his brother. They escaped, found a new stepdad...and then this new father figure was murdered.

Jocko Willink saw unimaginable horror in Iraq and lost close comrades in action.

Jim Rohn was a common farm boy whose life was falling apart in his 20s, finally got his act together, and went on to make millions. Then he lost it all.

Les Brown and his twin brother were abandoned by their mother, given up for adoption and grew up in poverty. He was branded "mentally retarded" in school and was given no hope of success – till he found his life teacher.

Life dealt them all a bad hand. They played it brilliantly.

They have crafted a winner's attitude and mindset

Notice how I say 'crafted'. A winner's attitude and rock-solid mindset are not something they were born with, or anyone is born with for that matter. These are constructed piece by piece over many years of facing difficult challenges physically, mentally and emotionally.

The teachers I've mentioned were put in a sink or swim scenario. They did the uncomfortable stuff over and over until they became comfortable. Pushing their limits grew their confidence. Seeing what they were capable of developed their elf-esteem, and it helped them naturally feel good about themselves.

By not taking the easy road, and working harder than everyone else around them, these guys steeled their minds and sculpted a whole new attitude that doesn't let them down.

Still a student of mastering your own mindset? Go find your teachers.

CHAPTER 20

Mastering Your Mindset In The Morning

It was shortly before midnight on December 3rd, 1999. A young American hotshot salesman was cruising along Highway 99 high on life.

The 20-year-old had earned more money than he'd dreamed of. He'd just been given a standing ovation for the best speech of his life. The girl he loved was with him, sleeping in the passenger side of his brand new Ford Mustang.

Life couldn't get any better.

But within seconds, it was going to get a whole lot worse. As the young man charged southbound down the highway at 70mph he'd no clue that his life was going to come crashing down round about him.

Coming in the opposite direction was a huge Chevrolet truck. It was doing 80mph – in the wrong lane - and the guy behind the wheel had been boozing.

The truck and car had a devastating, head-on collision. The young man and his girlfriend were sent spinning, before another car behind them smashed into the drivers' door.

The door pierced into the left side of his body. The metal roof caved in on his head. His body was shattered and, after rescuers cut him out of the wreckage, his heart stopped beating. He was declared clinically dead.

That young man is Hal Elrod. Miraculously, he is still alive today after being revived by medics and going through a long, drawn-out rehabilitation process. Today, Hal is a world-renowned keynote speaker, author and businessman.

But how did Hal manage to recover physically from such a horrifying accident that left him broken? How did he overcome the emotional trauma that flooded in as a result of the darkest time in his life? What helped him develop the rock-solid mindset and regain the mental strength that was needed to piece his world back together again...and then go onto achieve massive success?

His morning routine.

Those three words might well have underwhelmed you to a whole new depth of underwhelmedness. I doubt that's even a word, but you get what I mean.

Having a set morning routine with a specific set of habits may seem so basic and uninspiring to you. Yet implementing an early morning routine fed Hal's brain, nourished and strengthened his body, tested his willpower, built his resilience, and boosted his self-esteem.

Best of all: it helped Hal develop an unbreakable mindset that gave him the confidence that he WOULD overcome his darkest days and rebuild his life.

Following his amazing life turnaround, Hal travelled the world giving enthralling speeches about the power of his morning routine and published the best-selling book 'The Miracle Morning: The 6 Habits That Will Transform Your Life Before 8am'.

Hal preaches that how you wake up each day and your morning routine dramatically affects your success in all areas of your life.

The simple action of hitting the snooze button is not simply affecting that particular moment. Hal insists that it begins to programme your subconscious mind that it's okay not to follow through with what you're supposed to do.

It creates a pattern, a ripple effect, and can turn into a theme for a lacklustre, unproductive day.

This practice of implementing a set routine first thing in the morning before the day has even begun is shared by the sharpest business minds, the highest achievers, and the mentally toughest people in the world.

Those teachers I listed in the previous chapter – Robbins, Willink, Goggins, Rohn and Brown – they all have/had a morning routine. Each of those routines features various positive habits geared directly towards strengthening their mindset, influencing their mood, and building resilience so they can achieve their goals.

How These Teachers Start Their Day

Let's quickly look at the morning routines of a couple of those teachers to understand how they take charge of their mindset and get fired up for the day ahead.

Tony Robbins' morning routine, which he describes as 'priming' his body and mind, has become pretty infamous. Tony often talks about the importance of kickstarting his day with this specific routine that helps foster the right mindset and energises him.

Tony Robbins...

- Wakes up: between 7am and 9am.
- Takes the plunge: begins the day by jumping in his cold water plunge pool, or using a cryotherapy machine which drastically lowers your body temperature. As well as reducing inflammation in his body, Tony believes that nothing wakes your system more than a radical shift in temperature.

- Nutritional supplement: drinks a special formula of greens, vitamins, antioxidants etc designed to support his adrenals and keep his energy levels high.

- 10-minute meditation process: includes completing three sets of 30 yoga-based Pranayama breaths; a gratitude exercise focusing on three things he's grateful for; a connection practice sending love and good wishes to his family and friends; and visualising being successful in three goals in his life.

- 15-minutes of physical exercise: involving high-intensity training to raise energy levels and his heart rate.

Now onto Jocko Willink, whose morning routine is set out in strict military style. No messing around. While everyone else is sleeping, Jocko is "getting after it".

- 4.30am: Wake up. Three alarms are set incase one lets him down.

- 4.35am: Quick clean-up in the bathroom.

- 4.45am: Post on social media – usually of his wrist watch – to show his army of followers that he's up and ready for action.

- 4.50am: Grabs his gym gear – laid out the night before – and head straight to his garage for a weights workout that usually lasts an hour.

Being Disciplined – And Scoring Morning 'Wins'

Your mornings can set the tone for your entire day. That first hour can have a massive influence on your mood, productivity, performance…and how the next 15 or 16 hours are going to pan out.

When it comes to morning routines, I like to picture the whole process as scoring 'wins'. Your competition? That small guy that lives in your head and likes to bark orders, self-criticise, talk negatively, generally tries to fuck everything up, etc etc.

From the moment that alarm goes off, it's a battle between you and him. "Hit snooze…you need more sleep…it's nice and warm in bed," he'll tell you as you lift your head off the pillow, barely awake.

"It's nice and warm in here, I bet it'll be freezing cold if you get up just now," the mind-man says next, as you're still trying to figure out what day it is.

You glance over at your mobile phone. But, as that old saying goes, if you snooze you lose.

There's a better option. Give yourself a countdown of five seconds and, by the time you reach 1, throw the duvet off, swivel to the side, and spring to your feet. Do this quickly as physically moving your body briskly will briefly take the focus away from your persuasive mind.

You 1 – Small Mind-Man 0.

You've only been awake a matter of seconds and you've scored a win. Now it's time to quickly notch up another. Looking back at your bed, that creepy little voice appears again. "Check that state of those bedsheets...you're just up...you're bursting for the toilet...just make your bed later."

On the other hand, you can make your bed in 30 seconds and not have to deal with it later. You can make it really neat and feel good about that small accomplishment. You can then consider that another win for the day.

You 2 – Small Mind-Man 0.

After the flushing the toilet, that relentless little bugger starts talking louder in your head. "Wonder how many people have liked your new profile pic on Facebook?" he says. "You should really check your emails too...you might have received a reply about your job application."

Go down that road and you know what happens next. A quick glance on Facebook turns into a 40-minute flick-through of selfies, pictures of food on a plate, and unsubtle look-at-me cries for attention from people you probably haven't seen in a year.

If you log onto Facebook, Twitter, Instagram, or check your emails first thing in the morning, you're literally making other people more important than you. You're letting the stuff going on in their lives – mostly irrelevant and insignificant to you – affect your emotions and train of thought.

How about resisting the temptation of picking up your mobile phone till at least after 9am, prioritising your day and no-one else's, and then scoring another fine win?

Then you can move swiftly onto your morning routine, and strengthen your body and mind with a series of positive daily habits (physical exercise, hydration, meditation, visualisation...you decide). Then you can check off another 4-5 wins and the scoreboard will be reading something like...

You 7 – Small Mind-Man 0.

You see where I'm going with this? It's all about disciplining yourself with all the small things and, by doing them early in the morning, you build momentum.

Your self-esteem grows, a feeling of positivity expands, your discipline drowns out the small guy chatting in your head.

Ultimately, you build a stronger mindset.

Remember the Jim Rohn quote from the last chapter: "Every new discipline that we impose on ourselves will affect the rest of our personal performance in a positive way."

What's Really Going On In Our Brains

Whenever we experience even small amounts of success, or complete small tasks, our brain releases dopamine. This is a neurotransmitter – a chemical released in the brain which is connected to feelings of pleasure, learning and motivation.

Think about to-do lists. Whenever you complete a task and start checking off notes on the to-do list you get a bit of a buzz, don't you? What's really going on is that each time you place a tick on the piece of paper, your brain is spurting out more dopamine.

This is one of the reasons why I recommend to PT clients that they should always workout in the gym using a training diary. It means they can check off exercises as they're completed (increasing motivation) and mark up their performance in terms of repetitions and weights level (keeping track of progress – and cementing their commitment to their fitness programme).

When we feel the effects of dopamine so early in the morning after completing the beneficial habits in our daily routine, the positive feelings help mould the right mindset. We're also eager to repeat those same actions because it gets us to a place where we're being more productive and moving closer to our goals.

The world of work begins at 9am for most people. The more wins you can rack up before 9am, the stronger your mindset will become. I'm not hitting you with any of this new age, 'think positive and everything will be rosy' bullshit.

Staying disciplined isn't always easy. It's something I struggle with from time to time. But what is much more difficult is when you let the small disciplines slide, and they begin to stack up to bigger problems.

Boozing a little too much on weeknights...

Getting to bed late and hitting snooze too many times on the alarm...

Being late for work again...

A warning from your boss and having a crappy day at work...

Skipping the gym and then beating yourself up mentally for having no willpower...

Your sleeping pattern is all over the place, and then your hormones are thrown out of whack...

You get cranky and have stupid arguments with your partner...

You feel terrible and your head's "all over the place".

I could go on, but I'm feeling slightly depressed even writing about how that kind of scenario can play out. The fact is, most of us have been there and it can take a whole lot of pain to drag yourself out of it.

The end result of your body and mind being in the gutter doesn't just happen overnight. It's a domino effect after that excuse maker in your head takes complete control and your discipline with the seemingly-small things goes out the window.

A solid morning routine can help stack up those domino pieces again. It can give you a solid foundation for the most productive day. It can help you stay emotionally and mentally resilient when the brown stuff hits the giant industrial-sized fan.

You might be thinking to yourself, "what's all this morning routine stuff got to do with fitness and getting the most from my workouts?"

A lot more than you think. Firstly, by completing your morning routine and each small task, you're developing dedication and strengthening your commitment to what's important to you. This leaves little room for excuses or outside influences to throw you off track on what you need to get done.

If you can say no to excuses in the morning when you're tired and barely awake, then you can say no more easily to junk food.

If you can go through your morning routine and not skip any part of it, then you can complete a tough gym workout later in the day without skipping any exercises.

If you can drown out the negative voice in your mind offering up excuse after excuse, then you'll likely discover that you weren't performing anywhere near your best in your workouts.

BONUS RESOURCES

Download my 'Mindset-Moulding Morning Routine' free at: www.weighttrainingistheway.com/morning

CHAPTER 21

Welcome The Suffering

"Do what is easy and your life will be hard. Do what is hard and life becomes easy."
– Les Brown.

As the storm rushed in, the group of climbers huddled together preparing for the longest night of their lives. If they even survived the next few hours.

Xia Boyu and a Chinese national mountaineering team were stuck in the "death zone", not far from the summit. The mountain they were trying to conquer? Everest.

There was no hope of descending the mountain safely. Their only option was to stick together close to the highest point in the world – and pray the winter storm would ease off quickly.

It didn't. The gale force winds continued to batter Mount Everest and the team suffered sub-zero temperatures for three consecutive nights.

Xia generously and bravely gave his sleeping bag to a sick teammate. By the time he and the group got back to base camp after their unsuccessful climb, Xia's feet were numb with severe frostbite.

It was 1975 and Xia was aged just 25. His feet had to be amputated – or he'd die.

Then, in 1996, his legs were cut off above the knee after he developed a rare form of blood cancer.

Climbing Everest was Xia's dream and that dream had just disappeared. Still, he wasn't for giving up. With prosthetic legs in place and renewed ambition, the father returned to Everest in 2014. However, an avalanche killed 16 Sherpa guides early in the season, forcing most expeditions to call off climbing.

Xia returned the following year to pursue his dream, but the climbing season was cut short once again when a powerful earthquake struck, killing approximately 9,000 people, including 22 on Mount Everest.

Was it time for Xia to throw in the towel? Course not. The relentless mountain-lover was back again in 2016 and achieved what many people would consider unthinkable. Xia was back in the death zone – only this time disabled and aged 66 years old.

He was just 200m from the summit...then disaster struck. Harsh weather conditions swept in once again, making the final ascent extremely dangerous, and Xia was forced to turn back. He was heartbroken.

The following year, the Nepal Government imposed a ban on double amputee and blind climbers in a controversial attempt to cut fatality numbers. It was illegal for Xia and fellow disabled mountaineering fanatics to even attempt climbing Mount Everest.

Four failed attempts, losing his feet, being struck with blood cancer, losing both limbs above the knee, and twice coming agonisingly close to reaching the summit. Xia suffered for more than four decades pursuing his obsession. Then a government ban crushed his hopes and added to his pain.

Determined disabled climbers battled back, claiming that the ban discriminated against them. The High Court in Nepal overturned the ruling just a few months later.

For Xia, it was game on. In 2018, at the age of 69, the aging climber caught the attention of media all over the world as he set off on his fifth attempt to summit Everest.

At around 8.40am on Monday 14th May, Xia finally reached the top of the world. The first double amputee to conquer the mountain from the Nepal side, and the second double-leg amputee to reach the summit overall.

What's this incredible story got to do with your workouts? Why is a disabled, elderly Chinese man's achievement relevant to your fitness performance? What has scaling Mount Everest got to do with you achieving your health and fitness goals?

Xia Boyu's story is relevant because it teaches us three important lessons that you can apply directly to your workouts and pursuing those elusive fitness goals.

#1 It's possible – inspiring stories like this one show you exactly how ridiculously awesome humans can be. It underlines that no matter how many times you've failed at something, you can still dig deeper and finally get there.

Losing 60lbs, 70lbs, 80lbs or more and reversing type II diabetes? Finally being able to smash out the once seemingly-impossible chin-ups and pull-ups we covered in chapter 4? Getting in the best shape of your life and attracting the woman/man of your dreams with your new-found confidence?

It's all possible – when we lift the limitations we've dumped on ourselves.

Here's a personal example. I came across an article online a few years ago about a 100 push-up challenge. I rarely did push-ups. In fact, I avoided them because I wasn't very good at them.

I thought the article was suggesting you complete 100 push-ups within a specific time-frame, such as 10 mins. I was warming to that idea, but then I discovered that it meant doing 100 push-ups in one go. No individual sets. No rest. No messing about.

"NO WAY would I be able to do that…." was my instant reaction. Up until that point the most push-ups I'd ever done consecutively was around 30 – so 100 seemed impossible.

At the same time, the challenge excited me – and so I gave myself a two-week deadline to spice things up a bit.

I did push-ups every morning in separate sets until I reached 100 (i.e. 32, 28, 21, 11, 8). The aim was to complete more reps and gradually reduce the number of sets as I progressed.

Day 5: 100 push-ups in just four sets instead of five (35, 29, 24, 12).

Day 9: Three sets instead of four (42, 32, 26).

Day 11: Two sets (61, 39).

Day 13: I fell two short with 98 consecutive push-ups.

Day 14: I completed 101 on the last day of the challenge.

I'm not bragging as there are guys and women out there who are smashing out more push-ups without breaking a sweat. The point I'm making is that I thought it was impossible for me to do 100 push-ups in a row without any rest.

It seemed inconceivable...until I welcomed the struggle and got excited by the challenge.

#2 Perspective – Xia Boyu's story also gives you perspective, and this ties in once again with self-imposed limitations. When it comes to achieving their fitness goals, too many people are beaten before they even begin.

Doubts about what they're capable of. A lack of willpower. A half-assed commitment to training, their diet, and properly looking after their body because sometimes it's just "too much work".

Pushing yourself hard in the gym three times per week, getting your heart racing with a single sprints workout, and cutting out junk food is hardly work.

Getting to bed early, rising early, and implementing a 20-30 mins morning routine every day that's going to benefit your body and mind is definitely not work. It's called caring for yourself.

The real work is being done when records are broken. Real work is done when your mind tells you that you can't do another single repetition...and you do another three. The serious stuff is done when you feel so uncomfortable that the voice in your head tells you to stop...and you carry on anyway.

When you're working out and the weak-minded thoughts float in, just remember that there are people out there physically less-able but are still smashing it and setting new records every day. Keep that perspective and stay focused on constantly outdoing yourself, smashing your own records.

#3 Power – there's an irony in all of these extreme physical challenges, such as Xia Boyu's epic climb or David Goggins completing 17,000 pull-ups in 24 hours.

They break you down till you feel weak...and you become stronger than ever.

Why? Because when you welcome the physical and mental struggle, you become stronger and can handle the next one better. When you embrace the suffering instead of resisting it, the suffering diminishes.

Being dedicated to your training, your morning routine, cold showers, and maintaining discipline with your nutrition and small habits in your life gives you power.

All of it is like a training ground for your mind. Developing a rock-solid mindset through relentlessly pursuing your fitness goals means you'll be armed and ready to trod over the many other problems life can throw at you.

Forget Easy...And F@#k Realistic

It's time to lift the limitations we impose on ourselves. The majority of us are always cautiously gauging what we can and can't do, usually settling for the easier, more realistic option.

Forget easy when it comes to your workouts. Fuck realistic. Take the harder road...and embrace the suffering.

Hill sprints at 6am before a long day at work? Yes please.

A cold shower in the middle of January when it's snowing outside, and your mind's screaming "NO!!"? Go for it.

Attempting chin-ups at the gym and worried you'll look like a clown, feel humiliated, and the world might come to an end? Doing nothing is worse than failure, get on with it.

You develop mental toughness when you do what is tough. Welcome the suffering and see what happens next...

Conclusion

You've made it! By reaching this stage it's likely that your eyeballs have scanned over 43,573 words, 21 chapters, and one or two random stories you weren't expecting along the way.

For you, this is like finishing the marathon, swimming the channel, or reaching the summit. Actually, I'm lying. It's closer to you just pulling on your hiking boots and the massive challenge hasn't even begun.

Why? Because these 21 chapters are simply words. Those words must be translated - into action. Also, I'm not there to give you a swift kick up the ass. It's on you – and only you - to get things moving.

There are 21 lessons/lifestyle changes recommended within this book. They're all highly effective and have the potential to supercharge the results you've been getting from your workouts, particularly if you've hit a plateau with your training.

That alone is a sign that you need a different direction and should draft in new strategies on training, nutrition, recovery and taking control of your mindset.

Action is key, but action has an enemy...complication. We humans have short attention spans and we generally don't deal well with too many lifestyle changes at once.

A quick complete overhaul of your training, nutrition and daily habits is only going to overwhelm you, royally piss you off, and land you in a giant, steaming pile of manure called failure.

That's why a phased approach makes much more sense. First, I've split the fitness hacks into two groups: easy and difficult. I also recommend a three-step process for successfully introducing these fitness hacks into your life.

STEP 1: Take note of all the fitness hacks listed in these two categories

Easy Fitness Hacks

- Introducing anti-inflammatory foods
- Introducing anabolic superfoods
- Introducing power shakes
- Wim Hof breathing
- Quick workouts at home
- Intermittent fasting
- Avoiding artificial sweeteners
- Delaying your post-workout meal

- Supporting workout recovery with more sleep, magnesium, saunas
- Taking recommended steps to optimise your sleep
- Finding your teachers

Difficult Fitness Hacks

- Sprint training
- Cold showers
- Exercising in the morning
- Quick workouts at the gym
- Reducing/cutting out inflammatory foods
- Becoming a chin-up/pull-up champ
- Developing bigger, stronger arms
- Negative accentuated training
- Early rising and daily morning routine
- Welcoming the suffering in your training

STEP 2: Write down which fitness hacks you want to implement

It could be 12, 15 or 20 of them. You decide.

For example, you may want to skip building bigger, stronger arms (chapter 5), or miss out delaying your post-workout meal (chapter 14) because you get home from the gym late at night.

It's up to you, but obviously the more changes you introduce the better your results will be. Write your fitness hacks down in a journal/diary and then move onto the next step.

STEP 3: Introduce 1 easy + 1 difficult fitness hack each week

So that's two fresh changes to your fitness and lifestyle for the first week - and stick with them religiously. Then add in another easy one and one more difficult fitness hack the following week, do the same again the following week, and so on.

By stacking those changes on one another, you'll be able to keep building on those positive habits with fewer setbacks. This means you'll be able to maintain these fitness hacks more easily...and long enough to start seeing positive results in and out of the gym.

Remember that all the small disciplines matter, even if it's as simple as drinking a power shake every day. They're easy to do, but they're just as easy to skip.

Follow this process consistently until these fitness hacks become a normal part of your day. It'll quickly get to the point where...

Your body has adapted to intermittent fasting and you don't miss breakfast anymore...

Cold showers will still be cold showers - but you'll begin to love the rush of adrenaline and energised feeling they give you...

Getting to bed early on weeknights is a given...because you perform better, think clearer, and feel much stronger and healthier the next day.

Remember that each part of this book is as important as the other: training, nutrition, recovery and health optimisation, and mindset mastery.

Take one out of the equation and you'll struggle to build lean muscle, strip bodyfat and maximise the results from your hard-earned workout efforts. Take two out of the equation and you're going to get nowhere. Simple as that.

But be in no doubt that these Fitness Hacks work – and they have the potential to work extremely well for you. I'm sure you can guess what I'm going to say next...

For these fitness hacks to work, YOU have got to work.

I don't know exactly how you're going to react to everything I've laid out for you in this book.

You might be fired up to try out negative training in the gym. You might be feeling some resistance to implementing a morning routine, or you may have blocked out the painful idea of cold showers.

Either way, my response is the same: welcome the suffering.

Marc McLean

www.weighttrainingistheway.com

marc@weighttrainingistheway.com

BIBLIOGRAPHY / SCIENTIFIC STUDIES / RESEARCH LINKS

BOOKS

Tony Robbins, **Awaken The Giant Within** -
http://https/www.amazon.com/dp/0671791540/ 1992, Free Press.

David Goggins, **Can't Hurt Me** –
http://https/www.amazon.com/dp/1544512287/ 2018, Lioncrest Publishing.

Jocko Willink, **Discipline Equals Freedom** –
http://https/www.amazon.com/dp/1250156947/ 2017, St Martin's Press.

Brad Pilon, **Eat Stop Eat** –
http://https/www.amazon.com/dp/177511080X/ 2007, Self-published.

Les Brown, **It's Not Over Until You Win** –
http://https/www.amazon.com/dp/0684835282/ 1998, Simon & Schuster.

Jim Rohn, **My Philosophy For Successful Living** –
http://https/www.amazon.com/dp/0983841594/ 2011, No Dream Too Big.

Nick Littlehales, **Sleep: The Myth Of 8 Hours, The Power Of Naps, And The New Plan To Recharge Your Body And Mind** –
http://https/www.amazon.com/dp/0738234621/   2018,   Da   Capo Lifelong Books.

Shawn Stevenson, **Sleep Smarter** –
http://https/www.amazon.com/dp/1623367395/   2016, Rodale Books.

Vicki Culpin, **The Business Of Sleep: How Sleeping Better Can Transform Your Career** –
http://https/www.amazon.com/dp/B07CHZR33X/   2018.   Bloomsbury Publishing.

Dr Ellington Darden, **The Bodyfat Breakthrough** –
http://https/www.amazon.com/dp/1623361036/   2014, Rodale Books.

Hal Elrod, **The Miracle Morning** –
http://https/www.amazon.com/dp/0979019710/   2012, Self-published.

Dr Steven Gundry, **The Plant Paradox** –
http://https/www.amazon.com/dp/006242713X/   2017, Harper Wave.

Dr Mark Hyman, **The Ultra Mind Solution** –
http://https/www.amazon.com/dp/1416549722/   2010, Scribner.

Tim Ferriss, **The 4 Hour Body** –
http://https/www.amazon.com/dp/030746363X/   2010, Harmony.

VIDEOS

Ulcerative colitis and the Wim Hof Method.

https://www.youtube.com/watch?v=1n8WprOxl_g&t=7s

Fibromyalgia: Wim Hof Method.

https://www.youtube.com/watch?v=iFetmFua1iQ

Rhonda Patrick PH.D: How sauna use may boost longevity.

https://www.youtube.com/watch?v=eWKBsh7YTXQ

Vicki Culpin Ted Talk - A Wake Up Call: This Talk Should Send You To Sleep,

Tedx Exeter, 2018.

https://www.youtube.com/watch?v=VH268Xm2Czg

All Your Excuses Are Lies - Jocko Willink.

https://www.youtube.com/watch?v=6YjAk_l71Vk&t=37s

Joe Rogan And Mark Sisson On Post Workout Shakes.

https://www.youtube.com/watch?v=TOcxcCe8bbY

Paul Chek On Sleep, Cold Showers, And Parasites.

https://www.youtube.com/watch?v=0s5RRzPkj3I

SCIENTIFIC STUDIES

Ginger reduces muscle pain caused by eccentric exercise.

https://www.ncbi.nlm.nih.gov/pubmed/20418184

Anti-inflammatory activity of cinnamon extracts.

https://www.ncbi.nlm.nih.gov/pubmed/25629927

Relation of serum testosterone levels to high density lipoprotein cholesterol and other characteristics in men.

https://www.ncbi.nlm.nih.gov/pubmed/1998648

Relationship between serum levels of testosterone, zinc and selenium in infertile males attending fertility clinic.

https://www.ncbi.nlm.nih.gov/pubmed/23678636

Phytoecdysteroids increase protein synthesis in skeletal muscle cells.

https://www.ncbi.nlm.nih.gov/pubmed/18444661

Effect of Extracts of Ginger Goots and Cinnamon Bark on Fertility of Male Diabetic Rats.

http://www.jofamericanscience.org/journals/am-sci/am0610/111_3708am0610_940_947.pdf

Article 'How intermittent fasting might help you live a longer, healthier life'.

https://www.scientificamerican.com/article/how-intermittent-fasting-might-help-you-live-longer-healthier-life/

Fasting: molecular mechanisms and clinical applications.

https://www.ncbi.nlm.nih.gov/pubmed/24440038

Augmented growth hormone (GH) secretory burst frequency and amplitude mediate enhanced GH secretion during a two-day fast in normal men.

https://www.ncbi.nlm.nih.gov/pubmed/1548337

Favourable changes in lipid profile: the effects of fasting after Ramadan.

https://www.ncbi.nlm.nih.gov/pubmed/23112824/

Frequency and Circadian Timing of Eating May Influence Biomarkers of Inflammation and Insulin Resistance Associated with Breast Cancer Risk.

https://www.ncbi.nlm.nih.gov/pmc/articles/PMC4549297/

Fueling the Obesity Epidemic? Artificially Sweetened Beverage Use and Long-term Weight Gain.

https://onlinelibrary.wiley.com/doi/full/10.1038/oby.2008.284

Effects of the Artificial Sweetener Neotame on the Gut Microbiome and Fecal Metabolites in Mice.

https://www.mdpi.com/1420-3049/23/2/367

Measuring Artificial Sweeteners Toxicity Using a Bioluminescent Bacterial Panel.

https://www.ncbi.nlm.nih.gov/pubmed/30257473

Consumption of artificially and sugar-sweetened beverages and incident type 2 diabetes in the Etude.

https://academic.oup.com/ajcn/article/97/3/517/4571511#

Diet Soda Intake and Risk of Incident Metabolic Syndrome and Type 2 Diabetes in the Multi-Ethnic Study of Atherosclerosis (MESA).

https://www.ncbi.nlm.nih.gov/pmc/articles/PMC2660468/?_escaped_fr agment_=po=0.617284

Adaptedcoldshower as a potential treatment for depression.

https://www.ncbi.nlm.nih.gov/pubmed/17993252

Improved antioxidative protection in winter swimmers.

https://www.ncbi.nlm.nih.gov/pubmed/10396606?ordinalpos=1&itool= EntrezSystem2.PEntrez.Pubmed.Pubmed_ResultsPanel.Pubmed_Discov eryPanel.Pubmed_Discovery_RA&linkpos=1&log%24=relatedarticles&lo gdbfrom=pubmed

Voluntary activation of the sympathetic nervous system and attenuation of the innate immune response in humans.

https://www.ncbi.nlm.nih.gov/pmc/articles/PMC4034215/

Implementing a non-steroidal anti-inflammatory drugs communication bundle in remote and rural pharmacies and dispensing practices.

https://bmjopenquality.bmj.com/content/bmjqir/7/3/e000303.full.pdf

The National Sleep Foundation 2013 International Bedroom Poll.

https://www.sleepfoundation.org/sites/default/files/RPT495a.pdf

Professor Russell Foster Oxford University interview on sleep.
http://www.ox.ac.uk/research/research-in-conversation/healthy-body-healthy-mind/russell-foster

Effects of hour of training and exercise intensity on nocturnal autonomic modulation and sleep quality of ultra-endurance runners.
https://www.ncbi.nlm.nih.gov/pubmed/30389476

2013 Sleep In America Poll: Exercise and sleep.
www.sleepfoundation.org/2013poll

Acknowledgments

Weight training is the way. I love getting to write, teach and preach about it. Even better, I love getting to connect with readers all over the world every day, hear their stories, and help them out on their path to becoming stronger, healthier, better versions of themselves.

A special shout-out goes to the following awesome humans who are part of the Weight Training Is The Way tribe. They've all supported me in writing this book, and have helped shape the final version:

(Drum roll)…Reggie Baloun, Sharon Alfred, Janet Burton, Danny Conroy, Roger Chalke, Will Fairbanks, Joyce Fullbright, Luci Frye, Neil Harrington, Becky Holstein, Alan James, Elizabeth Kay, Rida Kennedy, Michael Kulinski, Manoj Kumar, Keith Lorino, Gill Marshall, Jay McConnell, Roger Mohan, Allison Regan, John Reinheimer, Denny Romano, Brad Smith, and Karen Wildridge.

Thanks to all of you!

About the Author

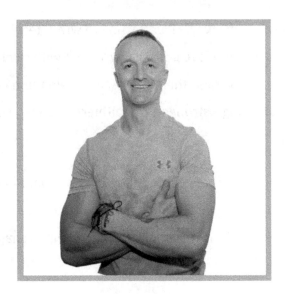

Marc McLean is a 36-year-old journalist and author who lives in the Loch Lomond area of Scotland.

This is the sixth title in his Strength Training 101 book series. You can view the rest at: amazon.com/author/marcmclean

Marc enjoys hillwalking in Scotland, playing poker with his pals who are not very good at playing poker, watching the UFC, road trips, eating out, and enjoying the outdoors with his family and friends.

You can connect with Marc here:

Website: www.weighttrainingistheway.com
Email: marc@weighttrainingistheway.com
Instagram: www.instagram.com/weight_training_is_the_way
Facebook: www.facebook.com/weighttrainingistheway

The Other Titles In The 'Strength Training 101' Series...

Book 1: Strength Training NOT Bodybuilding: How To Build Muscle & Burn Fat...Without Morphing Into A Bodybuilder - http://https/www.amazon.com/dp/B0774G2ZL8

Book 2: Strength Training Nutrition 101: Build Muscle & Burn Fat Easily...A Healthy Way Of Eating That You Can Actually Maintain - http://https/www.amazon.com/dp/B071NHHY6Z

Book 3: Meal Prep: 50 Simple Recipes For Health & Fitness Nuts - http://https/www.amazon.com/dp/B072J1SMCZ

Book 4: Strength Training For Women: Burn Fat Effectively...And Sculpt The Body You've Always Dreamed Of - http://https/www.amazon.com/dp/B0738K5ZJ8

Book 5: Burn Fat Fast: Ridiculously Effective Flab Busting Secrets Revealed - http://https/www.amazon.com/dp/B0744X4DLY

9 781527 237551